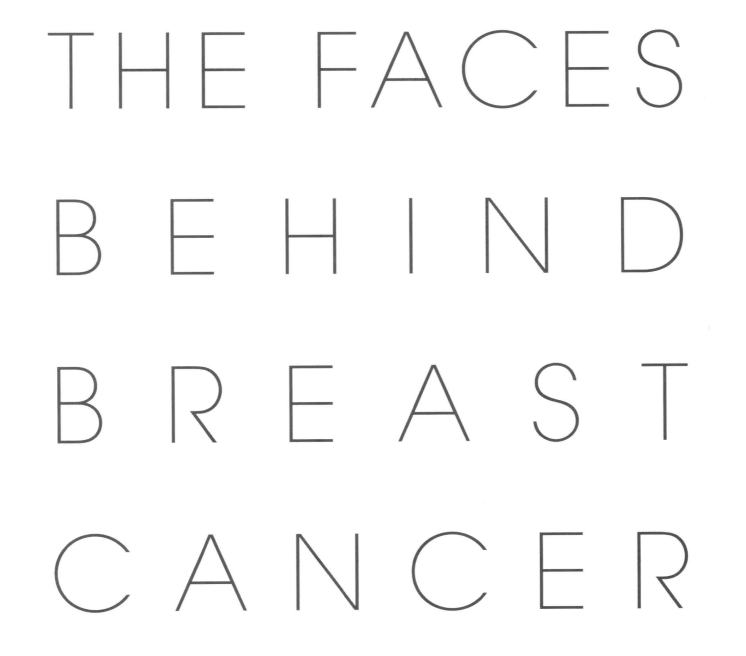

THE FACES BEHIND BREAST CANCER

This book is dedicated with love, gratitude and admiration
to my mother, Domenica Margaret Caruso, and
father, Saverio Caruso, M.D., D.L.F. of A.P.A.

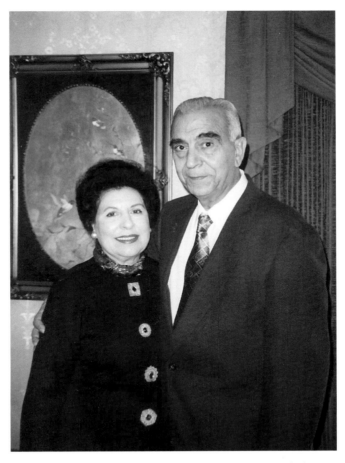

Family photo reprinted with author's permission.

Josephine
Caruso Sethi

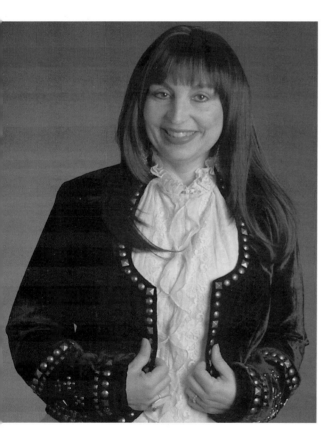

"Josie" was born in South Bend, Indiana, grew up in Ohio and is a graduate of Marquette University, Milwaukee. As a student, she was hired by a local television station as the first female technical director. She was one of the first women to join the Milwaukee Stagehands' Union. Following graduation, Josie was promoted to full-time writer and producer and produced a live, daily talk show, a weekly game show, children's programming, holiday specials, news promos and local commercials.

During the same period, Josie wrote, produced and hosted a syndicated radio show featuring female jazz and blues artists through The International Network of Syndicated Radio Productions, entitled 'Women & Blues.'

Before leaving Milwaukee, Josie assisted with the research and development of three successful cookbooks with author Sophie Kay.

In 1978, Josie was hired as a pioneer producer of Chicago's first all-talk format AM station. She produced a variety of shows dealing with current affairs, entertainment, health, politics and sports.

In 1988, Josie and her family relocated to the Boston area where she was hired by and later managed a local, cable-access station. She wrote, produced, and directed a variety of community-based programs for the town hall, school board, public service and special events. She also taught television production classes to adult and student volunteers, and won several awards for outstanding programming and community service.

In 2002, Josie assisted with research and development on a biographical book featuring singer/actress Cher.

In the fall of 2003, Josie was diagnosed with a rare form of breast cancer and underwent several surgeries and chemotherapy with unsuccessful results. She relocated to Houston for additional treatment at The University of Texas M. D. Anderson Cancer Center, including radiation therapy. In March of 2006, the cancer had returned and she had a bilateral mastectomy and additional chemotherapy.

Presently, Josie continues to undergo treatment while actively crusading for breast cancer awareness, education and advocacy. She is a member of the National Breast Cancer Coalition (NBCC) and the Houston Affiliate of Susan G. Komen for the Cure, and volunteers her time with local and national organizations, support groups and charitable events. She has a blog spot devoted to the cancer community: **(http://pinkcrusader.blogspot.com)** and a Web site as well: **(http://www.pinkcrusader.org).**

Josie has been married since 1979 to her college sweetheart, Tony, a management consultant. They have one son, Dalip, a writer and marketing representative and recent graduate of Villanova University Law School.

Jack Opatrany

Jack is an award-winning photographer whose diverse industry experience spans more than 16 years and ranges from fashion to catalog, and from people to national apparel companies. Jack prides himself on being cutting-edge, creative and able to bring out "the best" in a model or product through his photos.

A native of Cleveland, Ohio, Jack relocated to Houston in 1990 and immediately established himself as a top photographer on local and national levels. Among his achievements are top honors at the Art Director's Club of Houston Annual Show. Jack has been recognized for outstanding work on various projects and for donating his time to humanitarian causes.

Jack's portfolio includes people, stock, commercial and fashion photos. He lends his talents to magazines, celebrities, location portraits, model portfolios, miscellaneous products and high fashion.

Jack's commercial clients include Levi's; Nike; Continental Airlines; Compaq; Sterling Bank; Centerpoint Energy; Thomas Nelson Publishing; The University of Houston; the Houston Aeros; The Houstonian Hotel, Club & Spa; Houston Magazine; W Magazine; and Esquire, just to name a few.

Jack's celebrity clients include former boxer George Foreman, basketball great Sheryl Swoopes, Sen. Sam Brownback of Kansas and entertainer Bill Cosby, among others.

Jack is passionate about life and is a talented musician. Among his many personal interests are several charitable causes ranging from animal rescue, protecting the environment and, most recently, breast cancer education and awareness.

In particular, it is his love of dogs, especially his devotion to pit bulls, that inspired his recent pictorial, "Street Dogs of Mexico." This book is a fascinating collection of black-and-white images that capture the raw emotions and survival instincts of wild dogs as they freely wander the cities and towns of Mexico. Proceeds from "Street Dogs of Mexico," will benefit animal rescue and adoption.

For more information, refer to Jack's Web site:
www.jackophoto.com.

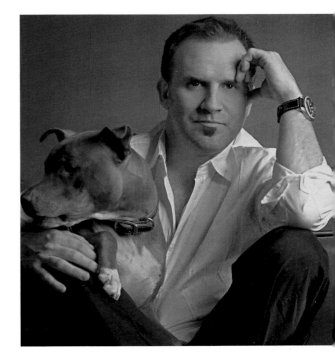

ACKNOWLEDGMENTS

We are extremely grateful for the kind assistance from the following organizations and individuals who helped make this book possible. We also express our deepest gratitude for all the emotional support of family, friends, caregivers and co-workers throughout the journey.

Emma Jacobs Breast Cancer Foundation

Alicia Dorn and Tim Elias of Alidotime Graphic
Design Studio (www.alidotime.com)

Rakesh Press, Inc. (www.rakeshpress.com)

Accent Insurance Agency

Bar Code Graphics
(www.sales@barcode-us.com)

Cellcosmet, a division of Cellap Switzerland
(www.cellap.com)

Intech Process Automation, Inc.
(www.intechww.com)

MAC Cosmetics (www.maccosmetics.com)

Marriott Westchase, Houston, TX
(www.pyramidadvisors.com)

Mr. Joseph Caruso, Caruso & Co. Fine Jewelers

Dr. Saverio Caruso

Dr. & Mrs. William B. Chan

Mr. & Mrs. Cheryl & Pat Donlin

Dr. & Mrs. James Geihsler

Mr. & Mrs. David Miller

Dr. Aldona Spiegel
Founder & Director of the Center for Breast
Restoration (www.breastrestoration.com)

Mrs. Rosemary Toscano

Dr. Sam T. Varghese

Dr. John Mendelsohn, President,
The University of Texas M. D. Anderson
Cancer Center

Physicians & Staff of M. D. Anderson
Cancer Center

DeDe DeStefano, Program Manager,
Development/Communications
M. D. Anderson Cancer Center

Lesley Icenogle, Special Events,
Development Office
M. D. Anderson Cancer Center

Sarah Watson, Senior Communication Specialist
Development/Communications
M. D. Anderson Cancer Center

Maninder P. Sethi, Business Consultant

Dalip S. Sethi, Legal Consultant

J.W. Cooper, Cooper Art Gallery
(www.jwcooper.us)

Cory Ezzel, Graphic Design Specialist

Chalon Fontaine, Fundraising Consultant

Gabbe Group, Public Relations & Media
Consultants (www.gabbe.com)

Brenda K. Hoffman, Fundraising Coordinator

Lisa Journagan, Event Planner, Connect the Dots
(www.connectdots.com)

Jean Karotkin, Photographer & Author,
"Body & Soul" (www.jeankarotkin.com)

OPA Mastectomy Products & Services
(www.opamboutique.com)

Hampton Pearson, CNBC Washington D. C.
Correspondent, Mentor & Friend
(www.cnbc.com)

Susan Rafte, Executive Director,
Pink Ribbons Project (www.pinkribbons.org)

Blane Smith, WABC Media Specialist, Alumnus &
Friend (www.wabc.com)

Peter R. Violand, Author & Poet, Alumnus & Friend
"The Man Who Brings the Waters"
(PRV9855@yahoo.com)

Jane Weiner, Executive Director,
Hope Stone, Inc.
(www.PinkHouston@sbcglobal.net)

Athena Laster, Professional Makeup Artist
(www.athenalaster.com)

Tanisha "Tee" Burr, Professional Makeup Artist
(www.makeupamore.com)

Shiwanna Archer, Assistant Volunteer Coordinator
M. D. Anderson Beauty/Barber Shop Services

Lilly Bui, Makeup Artist

Si Tran, Assistant to Jack Opatrany

Rosemary Barr, M. D. Anderson Network

Rosemary Herron, M. D. Anderson Network

Marsha Yeager, Coordinator SOS Support Group

Members of the SOS Support Group

Members of the Rosebuds I Support Group

Members of the Rosebuds II Support Group

Members of the Young Survivors' Coalition

Members of the Houston Chapter of the
American Cancer Society (www.cancer.org)

Members of the Houston Affiliate of
Susan G. Komen for the Cure
(www.komen-houston.org)

Participants

Family

Friends

Caregivers

Co-workers

TABLE OF CONTENTS

PREFACE

The following pictorial is a compassionate, inspirational and provocative book featuring male and female volunteer breast cancer patients in various stages of treatment and recovery, including lumpectomy, mastectomy, chemotherapy, radiation, reconstruction and remission.

Studies have been conducted since 1920 on the concept of body image and how it contributes to one's self esteem. When the breasts are altered or damaged by surgery, chemotherapy, radiation, etc., the mirror becomes the enemy. Many patients feel embarrassed, angry and/or obsessed. It can also affect interpersonal relationships and lead to isolation and depression.

This book is designed to give hope and inspire others to regain their self-confidence and improve their emotional state while learning to accept the physical changes in their bodies during treatment and recovery. Breast cancer survivors should never feel emotionally compromised or be defined by their disease.

Through the eye of the camera, we have captured a sensitive, yet realistic, photographic profile of a cross-section of cancer patients in a beautiful and artistic way. We have humanized the disease by exposing the faces behind the disease. The participants in this pictorial each share one common enemy, yet no two stories are the same, as told by their expressions and body language. These individuals are to be commended for coming forward with testimonies that resonate with strength, courage and conviction. They are all heroes as well as survivors. We thank them, we salute them and we pray for them.

— Josephine Caruso Sethi

INTRODUCTION

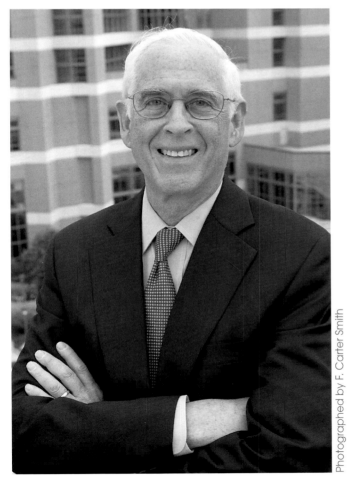

Photographed by F. Carter Smith

Photo provided by and reprinted with permission of M. D. Anderson Cancer Center

I am always pleased when patients and their families tell me what wonderful care they have received at M. D. Anderson. Many say that their initial fears of coming to such a large institution lessened when they walked through the doors and a volunteer greeted them with a smile and kind words. Other patients tell me that a passing employee noticed a look of confusion in their eyes and pointed them in the right direction or even walked with them to an appointment. I often hear patients say how apparent it is that their team of doctors and nurses personally cares about them.

Although I am proud of the care we provide and the scientific discovery that is such an integral part of M. D. Anderson, it's not our employees or volunteers who deserve the spotlight. The real heroes in the fight against cancer are the patients who wake up each morning determined to win that day's battle. The quiet courage in the halls and clinics at M. D. Anderson speaks volumes.

When I look at the faces of the people in this book, I see that same courage. The words they've written are expressions of the wisdom they've acquired while fighting their disease, but the unwritten drive, determination and hope that fuels each day's battle is also evident on every face. Their hope is our inspiration to eliminate cancer.

To Josie, who calls this book her "labor of love," I give a heartfelt "thank you." Not only has she created a phenomenal tribute, but, as testament to her compassionate nature, she has made 79 friends in the process. The pages in this book are not just stories — they represent lives, and Josie has truly shown the beauty of those lives as each person travels his or her breast cancer journey. We are deeply touched and grateful that she would put so much of herself into this project, all the while battling her own disease. Josie, thank you for walking the path with us, Making Cancer History®.

John Mendelsohn, M.D.
President, The University of Texas M. D. Anderson Cancer Center

SEASONAL

I

The season changes, and changes us
Until we turn and empty our hearts
Of energy, like waves
That burst onto mossy marrows of jetty
In storms along some coast
We'd half forgotten.

II

Over the city strange birds
Have been reported. They seem to be
Flying farther
South to a south we cannot imagine
Even in our dreams.

III

Over our favorite restaurant
The pecans ripen and rain
Terribly onto the roof.   It sounds
Like the world
Falling
To pieces.

IV

In this spell between the seasons
October's chilly light
Ignites the woods in manifold color
The leaves seem to be shouting:
"We'll endure! We'll endure!"

— Peter R. Violand

Reprinted with permission from
"The Man Who Brings the Waters" Copyright 1998

Participants

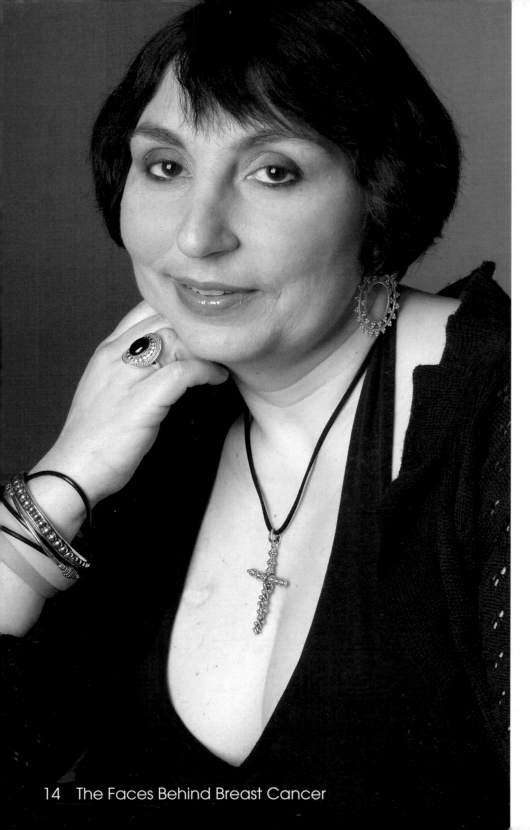

Miss Josephine

"Never Give Up. Never Give In. Never Lose Faith."

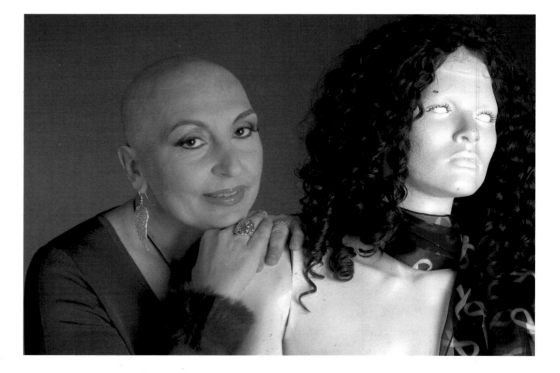

Martha

"I know I am stronger than I thought.

The cancer can take my body, but

it is never going to take my spirit.

I stay strong for me and for my child."

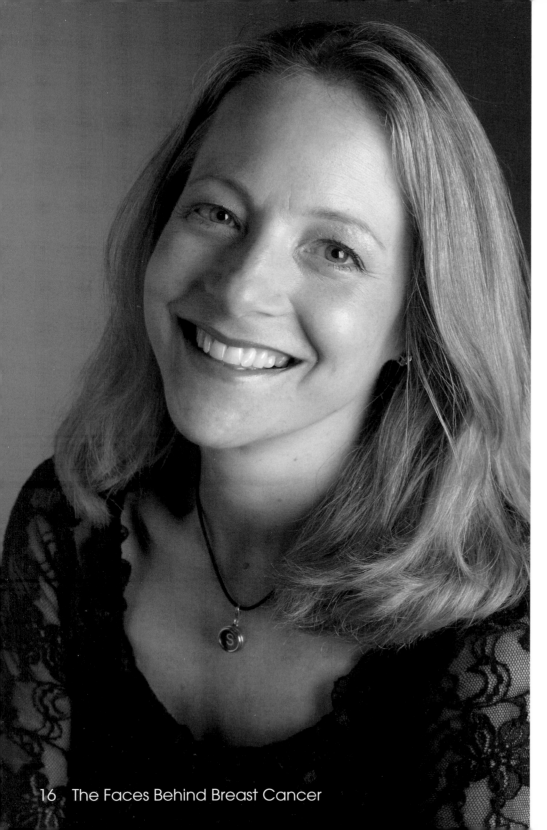

Susan

"Breast cancer: two words that changed my life forever. These words can be so devastating and tragic, but with most difficult situations, there is good . . . the silver lining in the dark clouds. For me, the journey with breast cancer has taken me to many wonderful places, both internal and external. My relationships have been made stronger, and I have met many fabulous people who share this common bond. I have found an inner strength and a passionate direction that would otherwise have lain dormant. I have been able to make my personal story grow and become my powerful professional story through the many areas of the breast cancer community that I am involved with, especially as the executive director of the Pink Ribbons Project, Dancers in Motion against Breast Cancer.

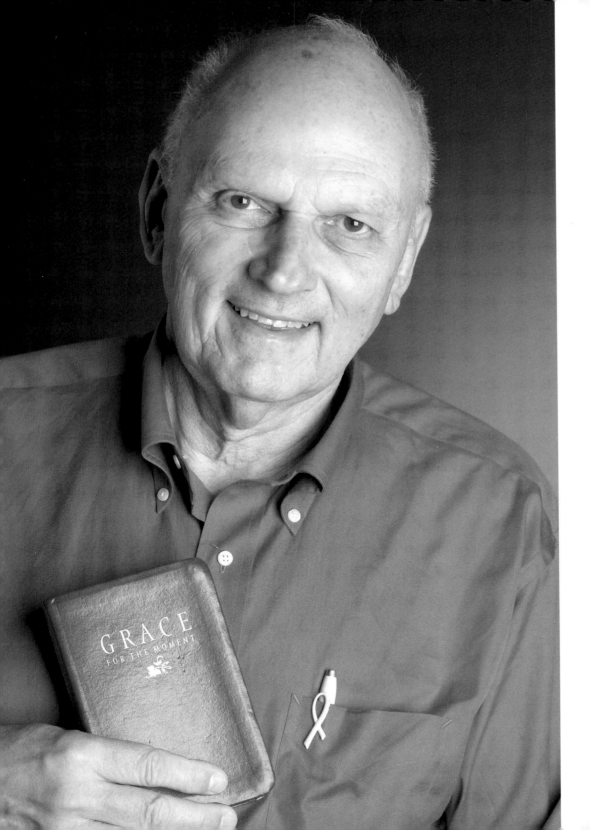

John

"I know that many people are surprised when I say that having breast cancer was a big positive in my life, but it was. Cancer is nothing that anyone would volunteer for, but I personally learned oh so very much about the love and care from my wife, family and friends. This, coupled with amazing medical care and especially God's guiding Light, totally overwhelmed any negatives."

Janice

"When the world says
GIVE UP,

hope steps in and says

try one more time."

HOPE

Janice & Rogers

Melanie

"I now have a different outlook on life. I never take anything for granted anymore. I have become a stronger person. It has made me become closer to the Lord."

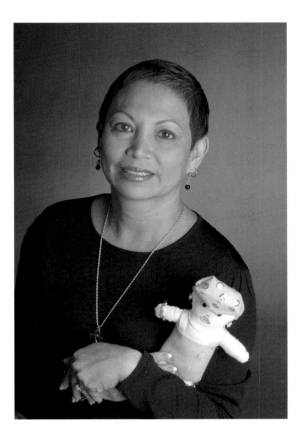

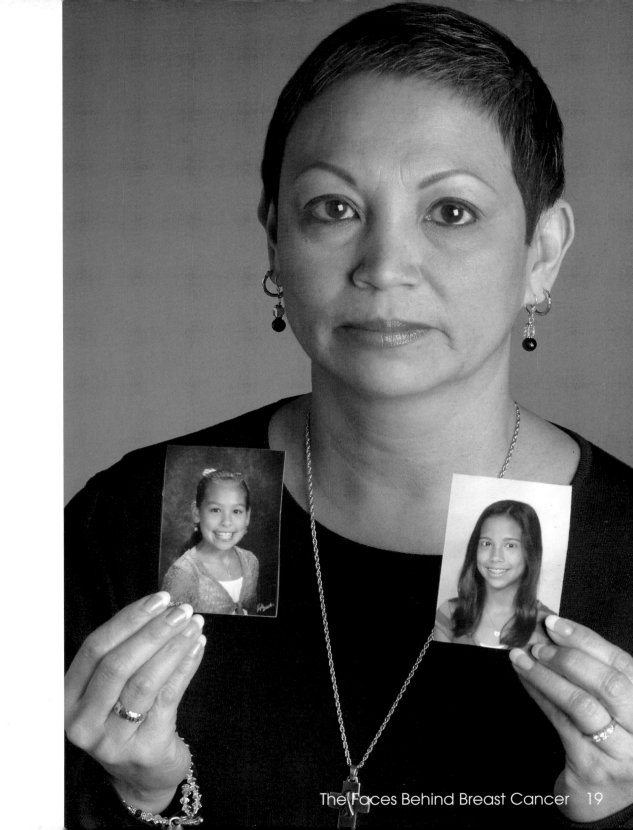

Laura

"Breast cancer has made me understand courage. I don't feel like a brave person. I've come to understand that courage is sometimes just, putting one foot in front of the other. During this time, I held onto a Camus quote: 'In the middle of my winter, I discovered that in me, there was an invincible summer.'"

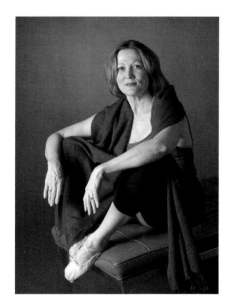

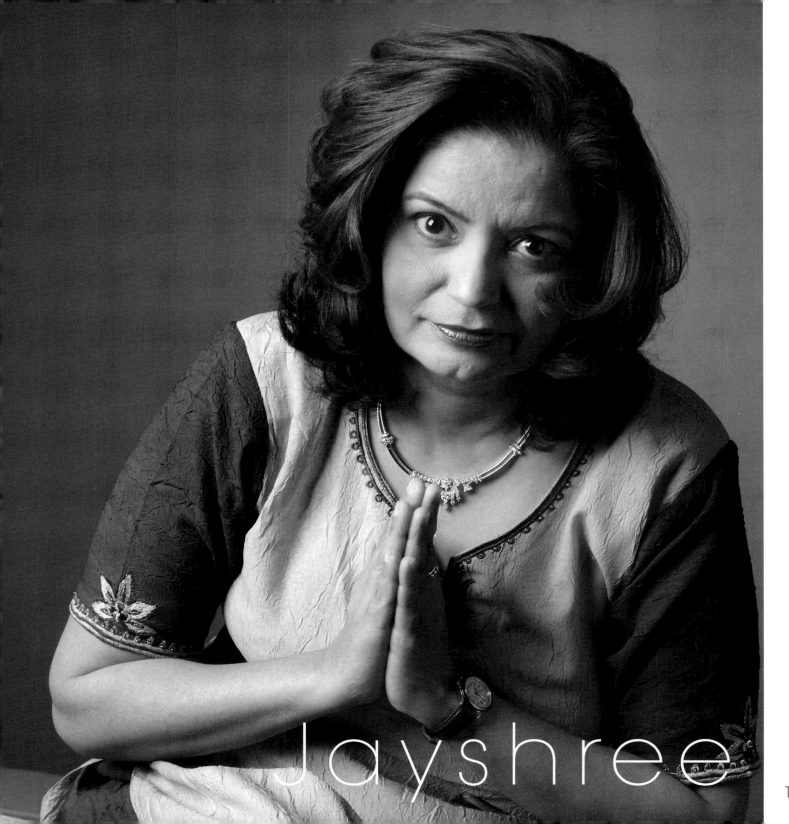

Jayshree

"Breast cancer was a challenge for me. I was shocked when I found out but faced it happily with prayer. If God had given me this challenge, He would also give me the strength to fight it out. As a parent, with two small children, I tell all those who have this disease to bravely and boldly fight it out. You will pass this journey with flying colors!"

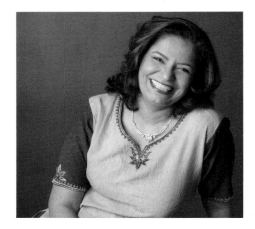

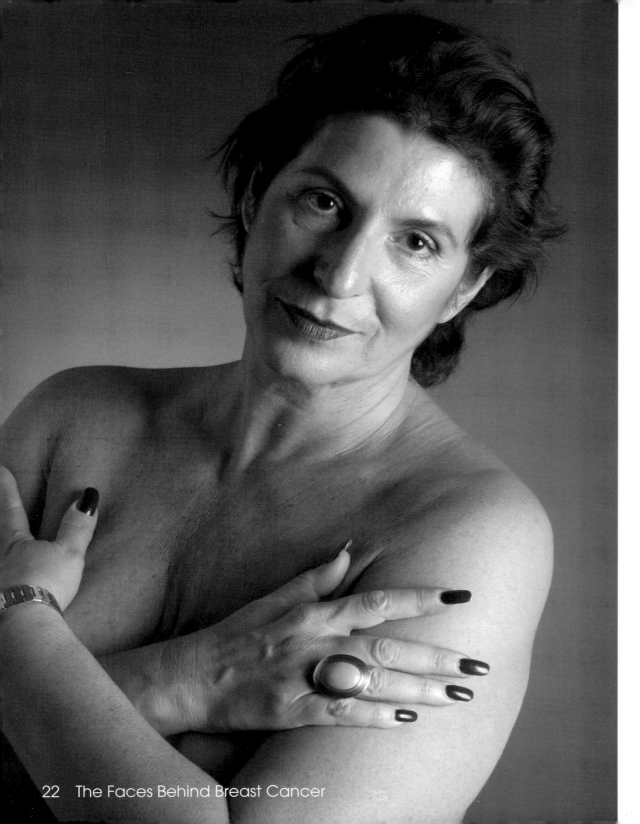

Emma

"My experience with breast cancer made me very conscious of how precious life is, and I do not take things for granted anymore. I also realize the importance of good health and how great it is to feel good!"

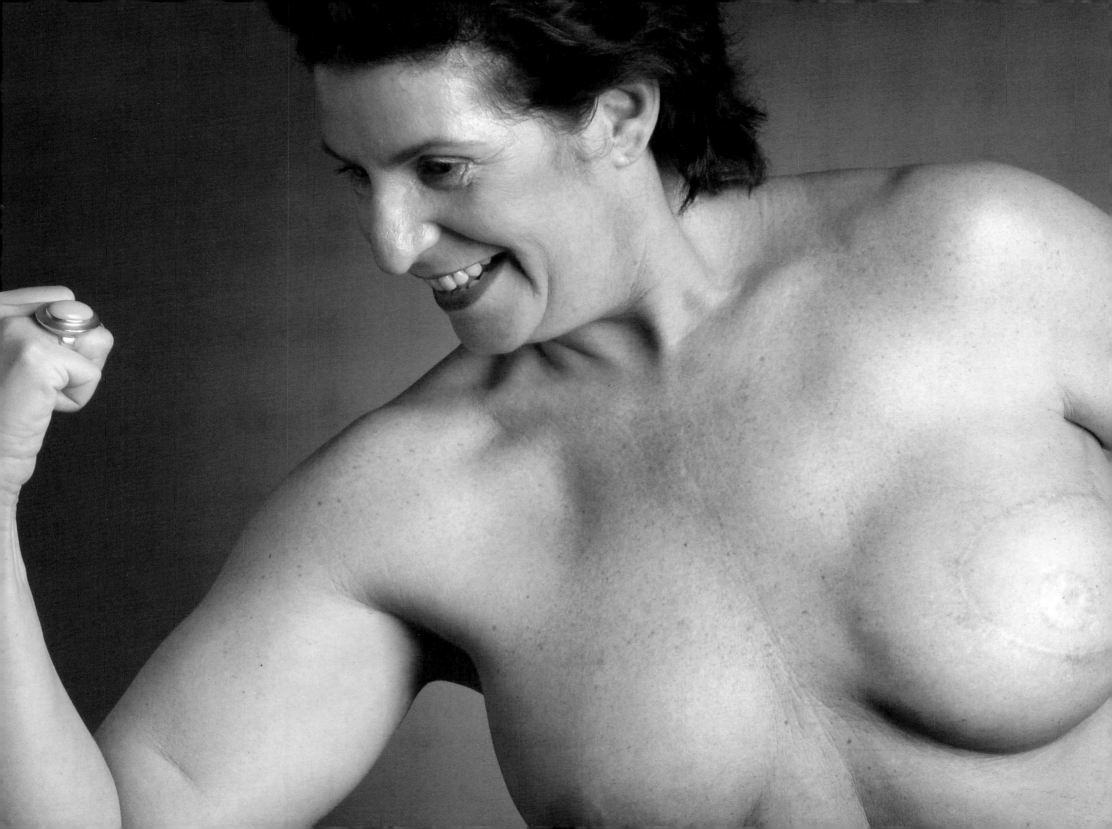

Mary

"Thank the Good Lord above that modern technology detected my breast cancer at the earliest stage possible. After a bilateral mastectomy and reconstruction, my surgical oncologist, Dr. Eva Singletary, from M. D. Anderson Cancer Center, said, 'Consider this a blip on the radar screen of your life. I'll see you in one year!' Being a breast cancer survivor is not a sorority you rush to sign up for; however, it is a sisterhood that transforms your life forever!"

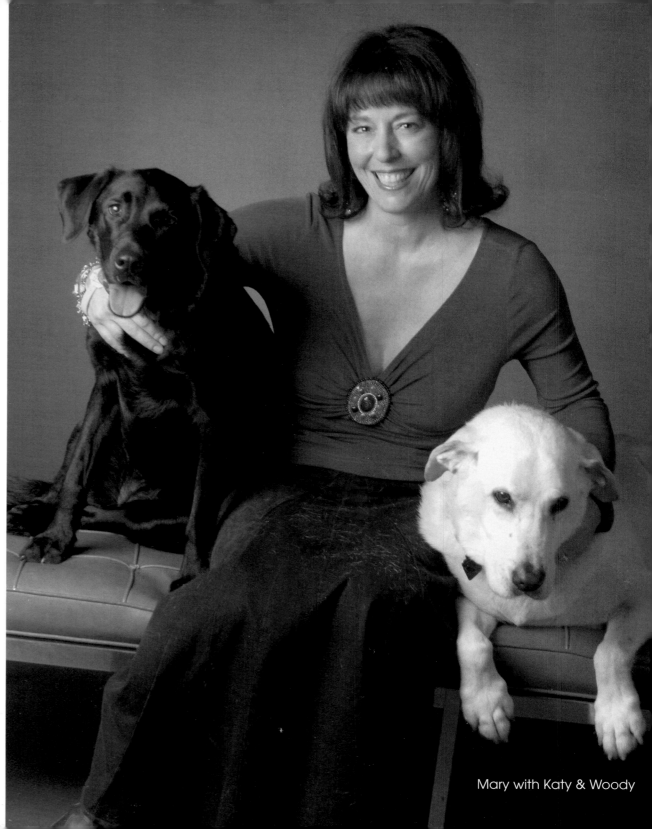

Mary with Katy & Woody

Jackie

"Cancer brought me into a whole different world where I've made friends with people I probably would have never met. We have bonded through our journey of cancer and also lost friends to this horrible disease, which is always devastating."

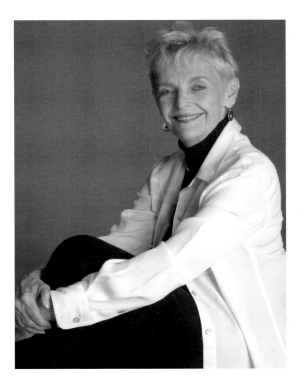

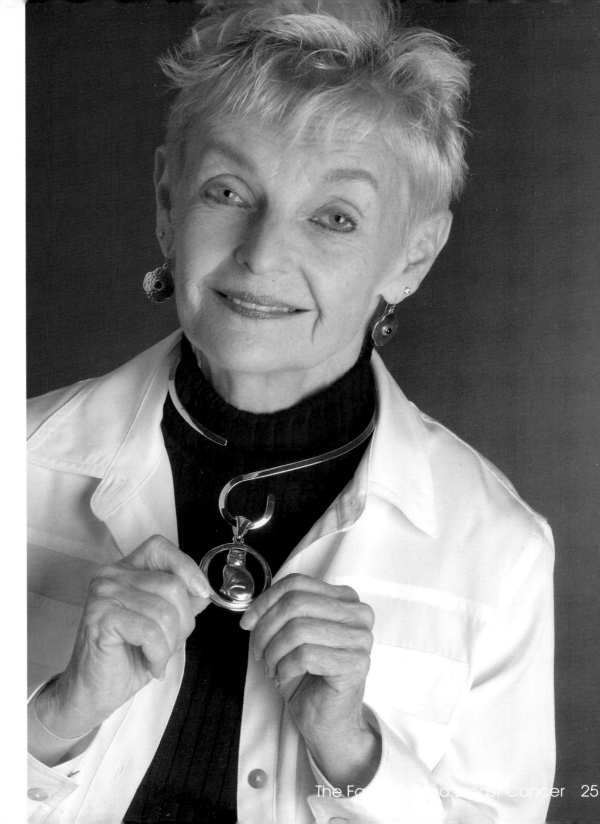

Carolyn

"Once I heard the words 'breast cancer,' all of life's little details that seemed so important five minutes ago became one big blur. The only clarity was my husband and our daughters. Their love is what has made me so strong during this fight. Their love is why I will win."

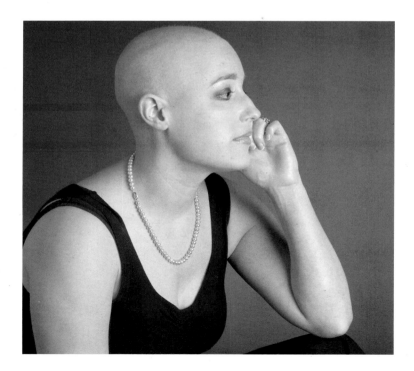

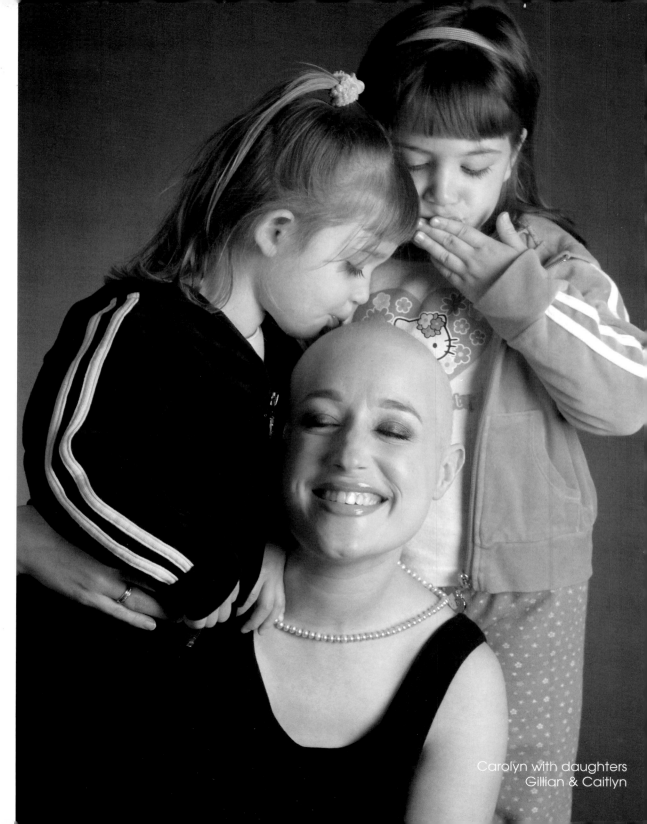

Carolyn with daughters
Gillian & Caitlyn

Margaret

"Facing cancer is a daunting proposition. For me, getting through it took purposeful determination, a strong will and the love and support of family and friends. Sometimes, though, all it takes to keep going is a warm hug."

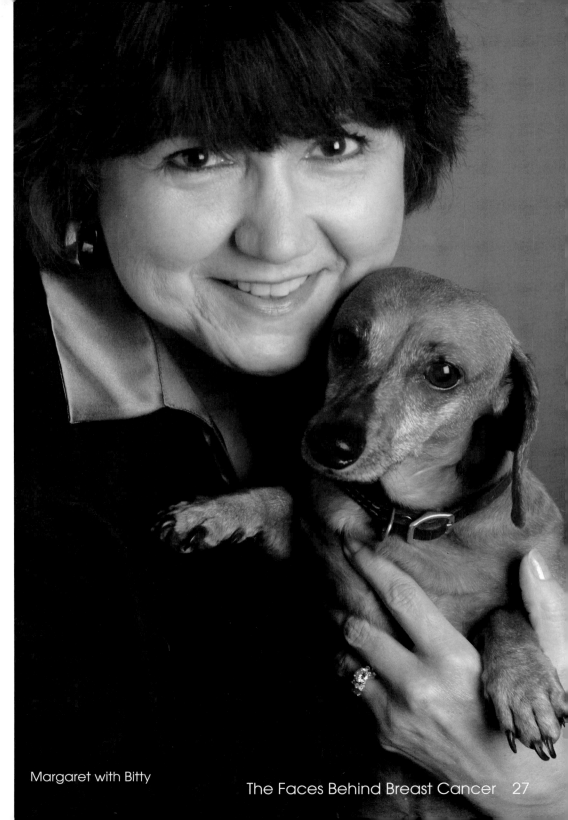

Margaret with Bitty

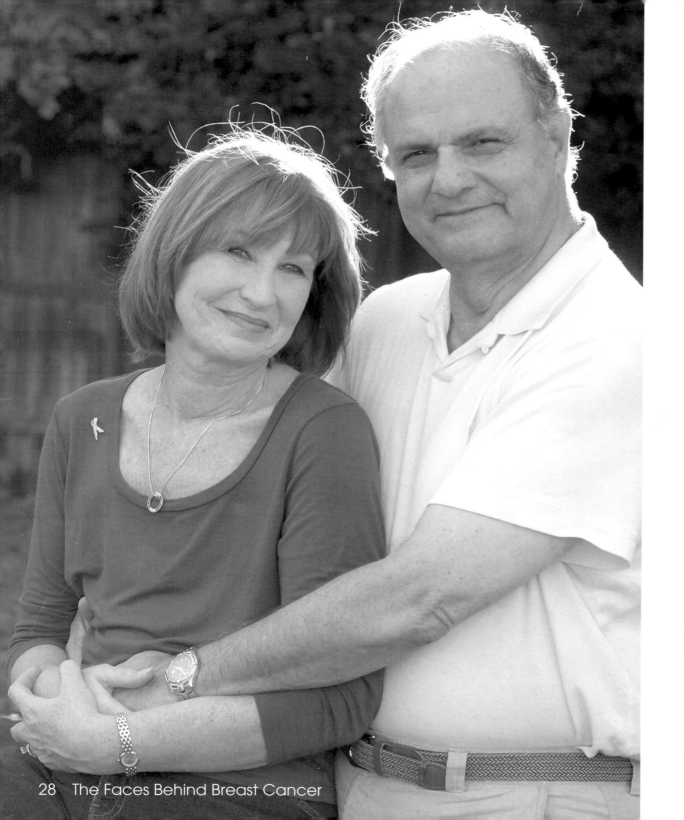

Kelly Jo

"I have gained far more from having breast cancer than I ever lost. I am not missing anything. LIVE, LOVE, LAUGH!"

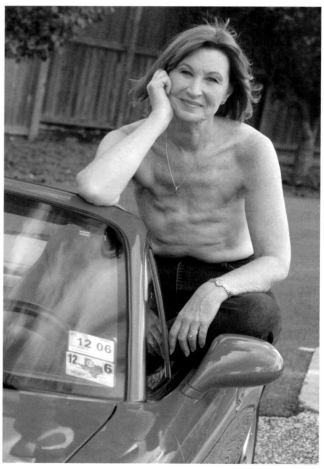

Kelly Jo & Norm

Leslie

For the first months, crying, and with big tears, was cathartic. I also found great comfort in a breast cancer support group. And, after eleven years, I keep going back to that wonderful group of women, gaining inspiration by supporting the newly diagnosed. Also, at 50, I bought my first pair of running shoes. There have not been any races, but I just try to wear out a pair of shoes every now and then. My life is not a marathon—it is about treasuring TODAY.

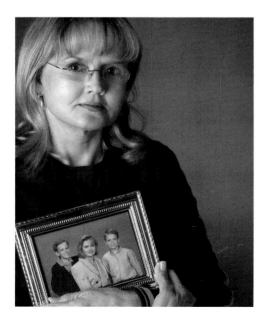

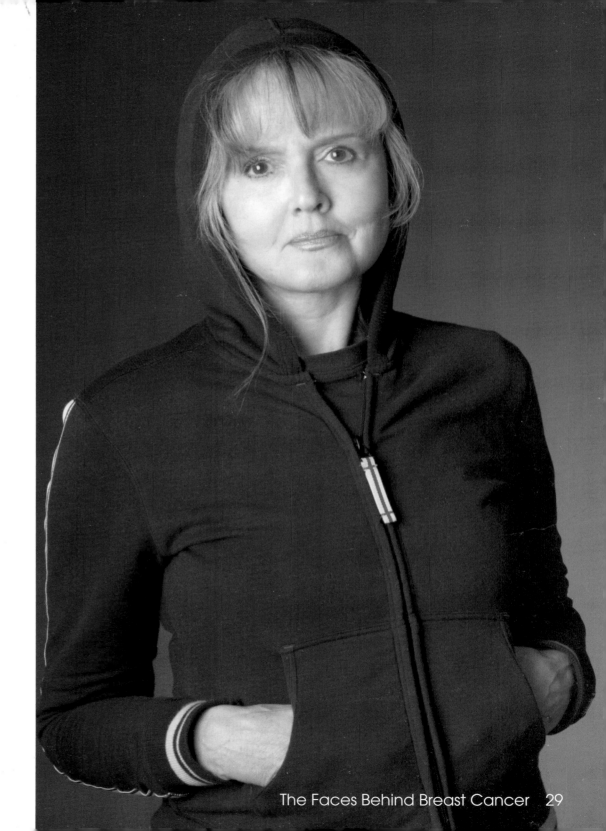

Judy

"With my cancer diagnosis, I literally felt I was going to war. Through God's grace, the support of my family and friends, and the expertise of my oncologist, surgeons and staff at M. D. Anderson, I survived the many battles and made it back from the war zone. If I made it, you can too! So get your mammograms routinely."

Judy with daughters
Nona & Mimi

Rosemary

"My cancer experience has shown me that our relationships with God, family, friends and acquaintances are what really matters. My faith in God, the love and support of my husband and family, along with the care and concern of friends, carried me through diagnosis, treatment and survivorship. I am blessed!"

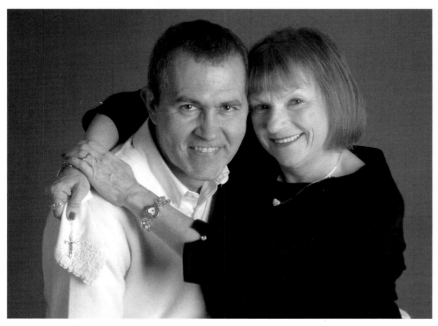

Rosemary & Don

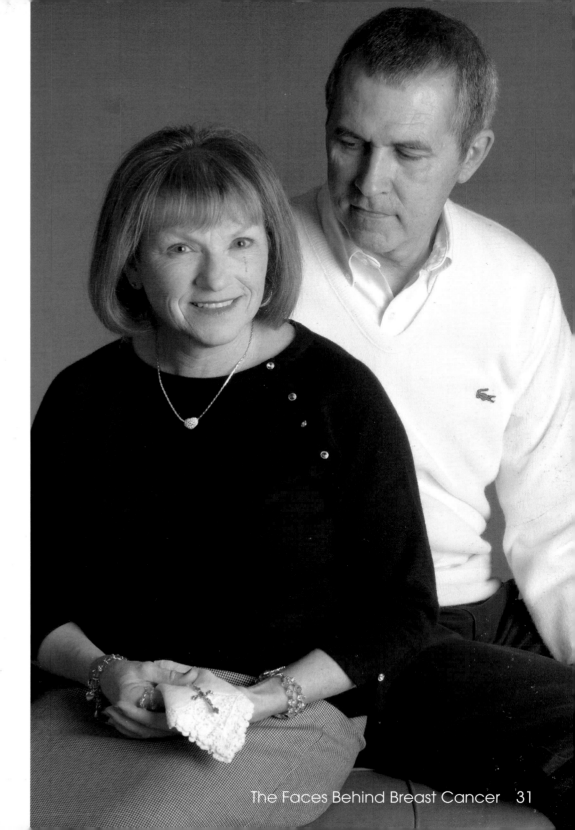

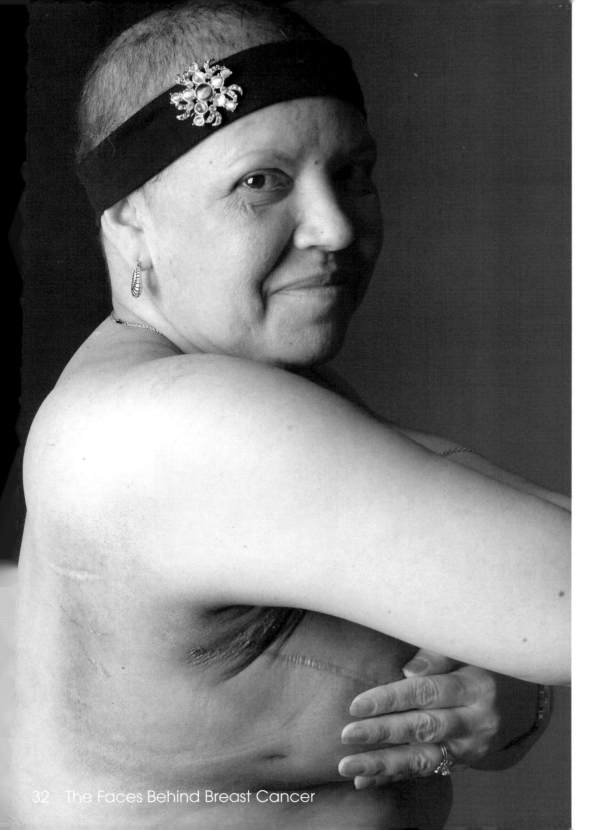

Argelia

"Determination and Optimism equal Survival (the Scorpion Way). Cancer is a minor set-back in lifestyle, but it is only temporary. We should appreciate life as we live today and not worry about tomorrow."

Stephanie

"On my first day of testing at M. D. Anderson Cancer Center,

I met a young woman wearing a turban who told me that

her hair was starting to grow back after chemotherapy. She

laughed and said it must be a sign of spring. I now also view

my new hair not only as a sign of spring, but also one of

rebirth. Breast cancer has been a difficult journey at times,

but I discovered that I possess a strength I never knew I had.

I am treating my diagnosis date as my Survivor Birthday and

will celebrate each year to come."

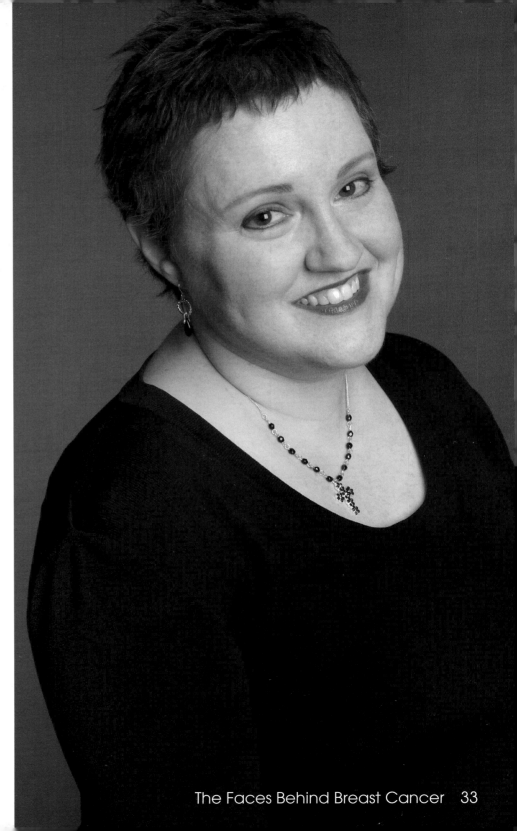

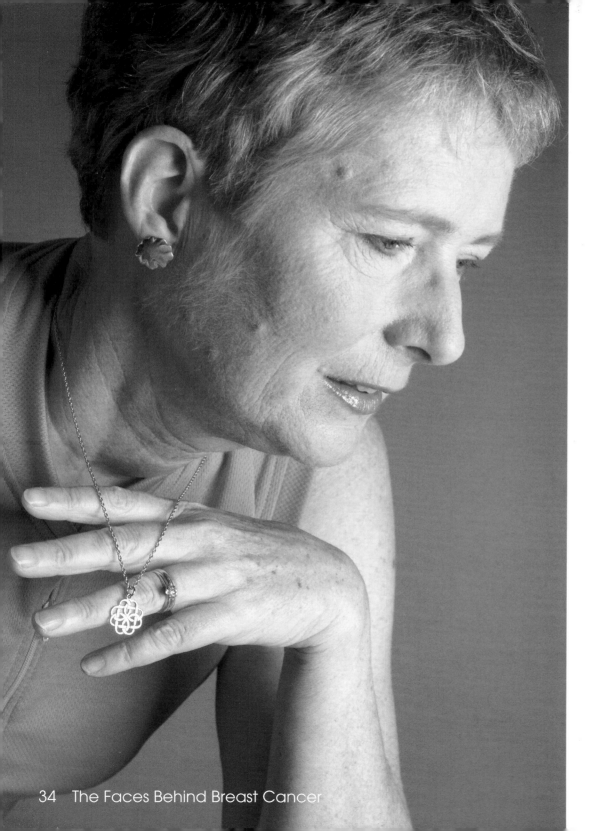

Barbara

"Living with breast cancer is now a constant for me. My goal is not to lose my identity, not to let cancer take away the active, involved person I have always been.

My family and friends have always been the

center of my life. Cancer will have to stand aside

for them."

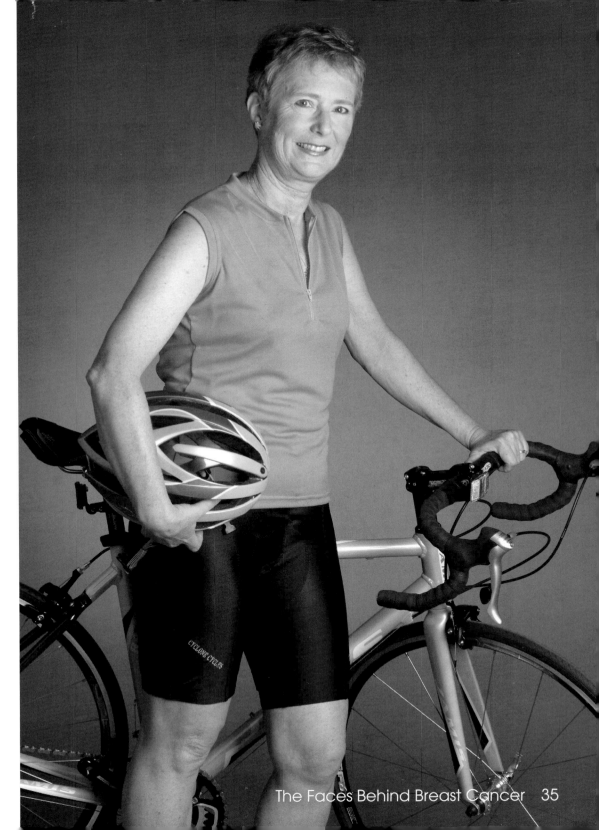

Angie

A Survivor's Creed

I am a Survivor.
Today I choose to live
with strength and courage.
I will be thankful for the beauty of
the ordinary things that surround me.
I may have a weakened body,
but I have an inspired spirit.
I will not fear the future,
I will not fear the present.
I will live in the moment.
I choose to believe that
statistics don't apply to me.
I am my own statistic.
I will build an
extraordinary life,
so no matter when
I leave this earth;
I will leave a legacy of love,
and of strength, and of courage.
I will not become bitter because of
my circumstances. I will allow them to
shape me, and make me a better person.
I will overcome! I am a Survivor!

©2005 Angela Elliott - Inflammatory Breast Cancer Survivor
www.survivorscreed.com

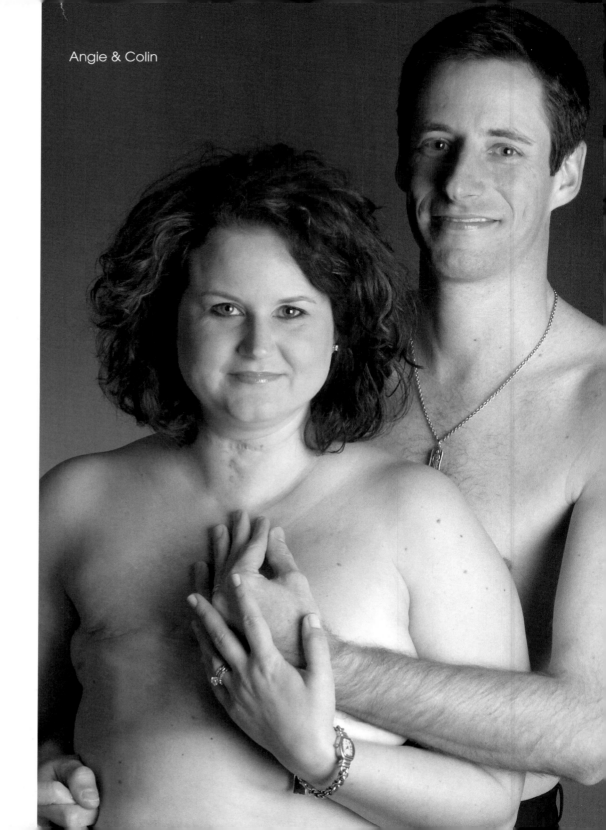

Angie & Colin

Mary

"Breast cancer has given me a new birth on life . . . to see things in a new way and to not worry about the things I used to worry about. I also have a better appreciation of things that I did not used to have."

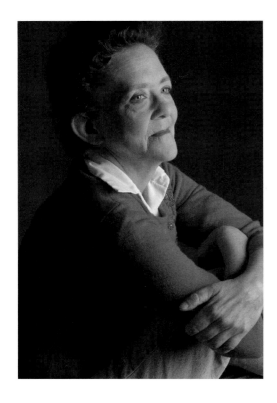

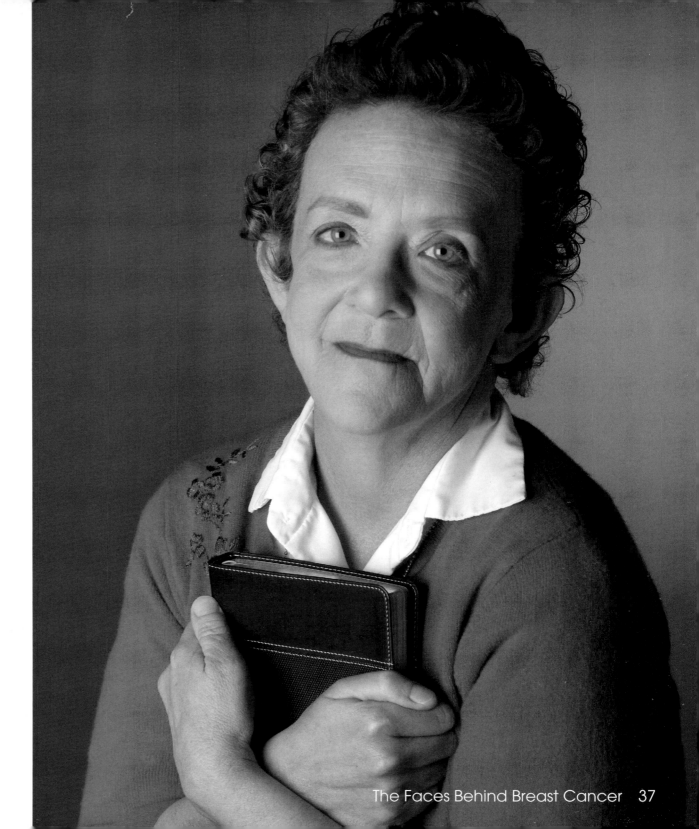

Kristi

"Breast cancer has taken a lot from my family. My grandmother eventually lost an arm due to complications from breast cancer. My mother lost her life to breast cancer. I lost a part of my youth to breast cancer when I was diagnosed at 32. But breast cancer has also given me beautiful gifts. I have met some of the strongest and most inspiring women who are fellow breast cancer survivors. I have learned to appreciate life and how fragile and precious it is. I have found purpose in my life through helping other young women with breast cancer. Breast cancer has shaped who I am today. My daughter once observed that breast cancer is our family legacy. More than anything, I don't want my daughter to have a family legacy defined by disease, but instead, by action, courage and survival.

Kristi with daughter Madison

Sandra

"The value of a person lies not in the physical assets or charm. The true self is what lies within the heart. The grace and mercies of God, along with cherished friends, make the journey filled with precious moments. Now is the time to live in the moment. Living 100 percent will capture the moment of now. Know the gift of life and the gift of yourself. Live all the days filled with intense love, joy, hope and faith."

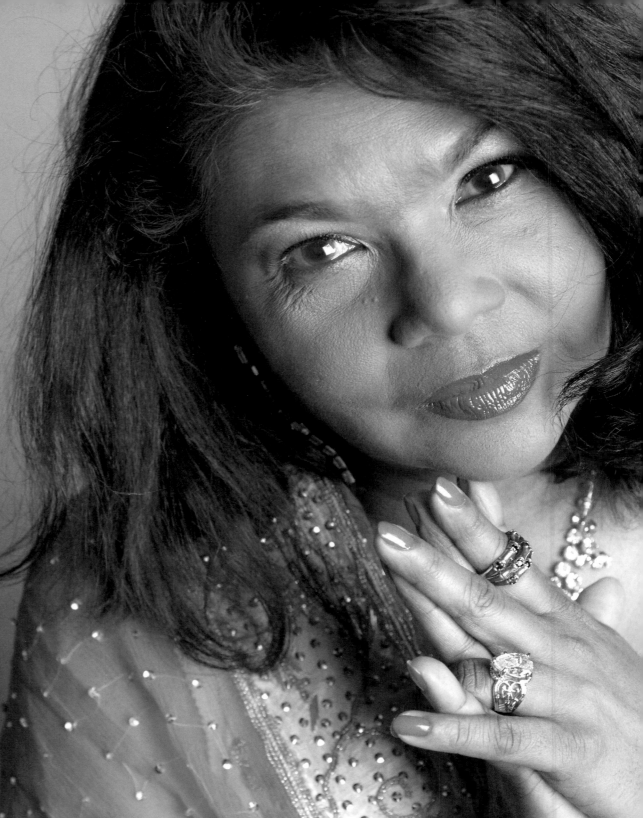

Cheryl

"At 56, I'd decided to change my life, to stop waiting for the 'perfect' time for things. So, I finished my undergraduate degree (begun 38 years earlier!), moved to a new part of town and took a new job in a different field. Then, fate handed me a really urgent mandate for change: breast cancer. Two years later, minus a breast but more alive than ever, I've made the most fundamental change of all by choosing to live in the now and to be truly present in each day of my life, for myself and those I love. Life is sweet, and I refuse to waste another minute worrying about a possible future that may never come, or waiting for the right time. The right time is now. Work. Create. Grow. Give."

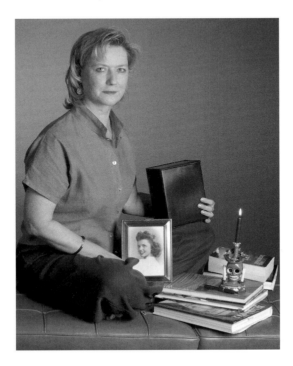

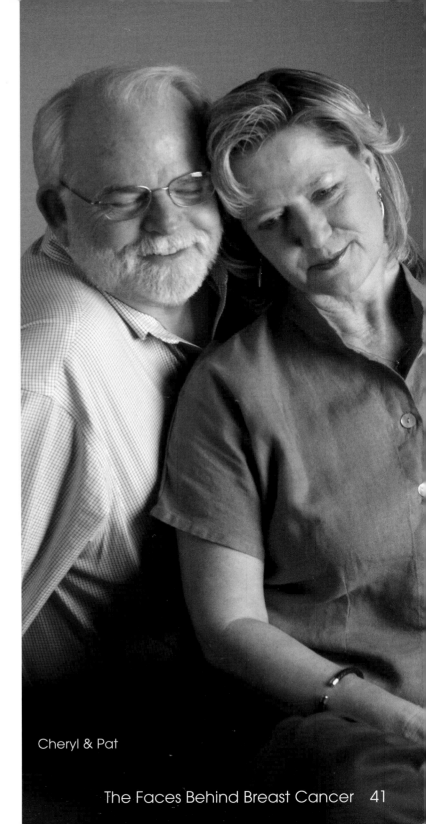

Cheryl & Pat

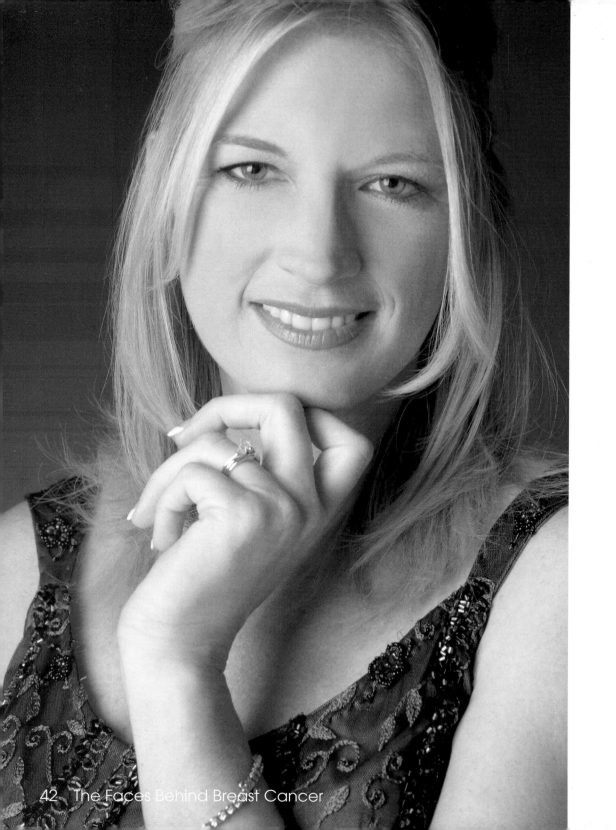

Cindy

"You never know how much strength you have until you're faced with the greatest challenges of your life. You also never realize the beauty people possess until they are met with the opportunity to serve others. Through having cancer, along with some other challenges I've had in my life, I have learned that I am strong and that there is something beautiful inside of everyone."

Destini

"Breast cancer has affected so much and so many things in my life: new breasts, new outlook on life, new appreciation for motherhood. Through it all, you have moments of great sadness and great happiness, but the gift is when, with true clarity, you can sit back and thank God for this journey because everything after treatment becomes a piece of cake. When the dust settles, you have become this improved, confident, thankful, grateful human being that God intended you to be . . . and you love life more for it."

Destini with daughters Indya & Imry

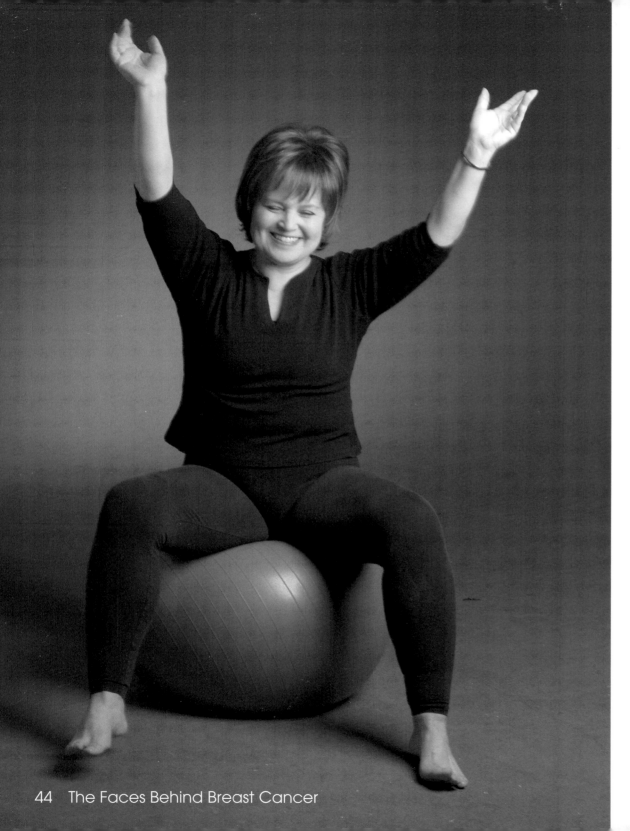

Becky

"Like any major life illness, breast cancer instantly prioritizes each aspect of your life. Now you innately know what's important. What was a huge problem before is now a minor inconvenience."

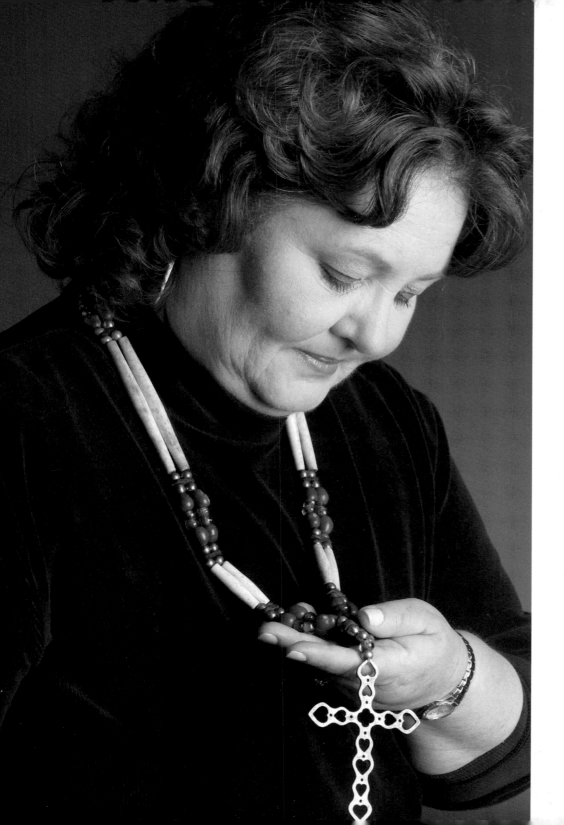

Elizabeth

"God has given me a wonderful journey and so many lessons to learn. Cancer has taught me fear, but more important, it has also taught me about the love of family and friends, compassion, healing care, powerful prayers and courageous women. God has blessed me on this journey."

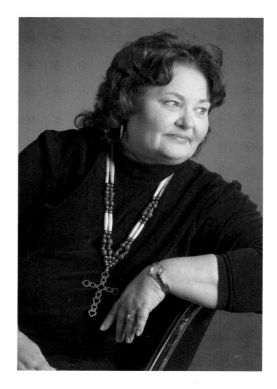

Wendy

"Breast cancer has taught me that happiness can exist simultaneously with pain and fear. I have developed relationships with myself and others that are deeper and more meaningful than ever before. I have learned that inward beauty is much more important than looking at the outward scars that breast cancer has created."

Wendy & daughter Kendall

Barbara

"Cancer gave me the opportunity to gain an understanding of myself and to realize how much I have to offer the world. I finally like myself!"

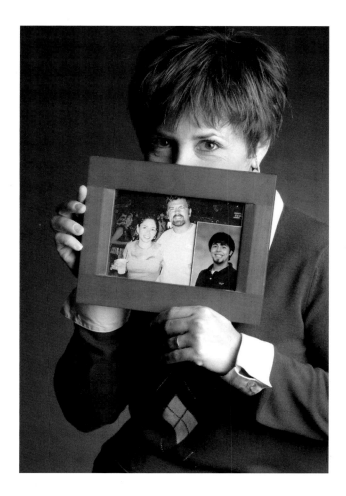

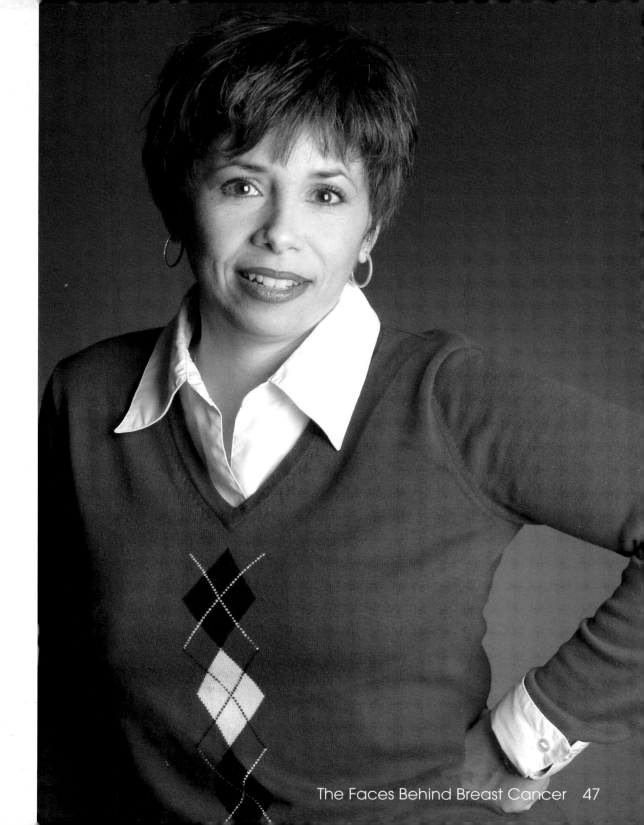

Britt

"Breast cancer has made me more appreciative of life's little things. It has not only affected me, but also all of those who love me, such as my husband. I was diagnosed just three weeks prior to our wedding in March 2006."

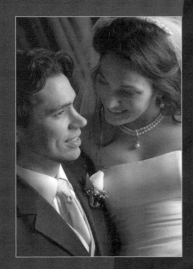

Ann
Nette

"The only good thing about having cancer is that you have so many people pray-
ing for you . . . including many strangers
remembering me in their prayers. It is such
a powerful experience."

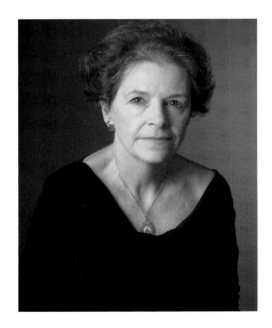

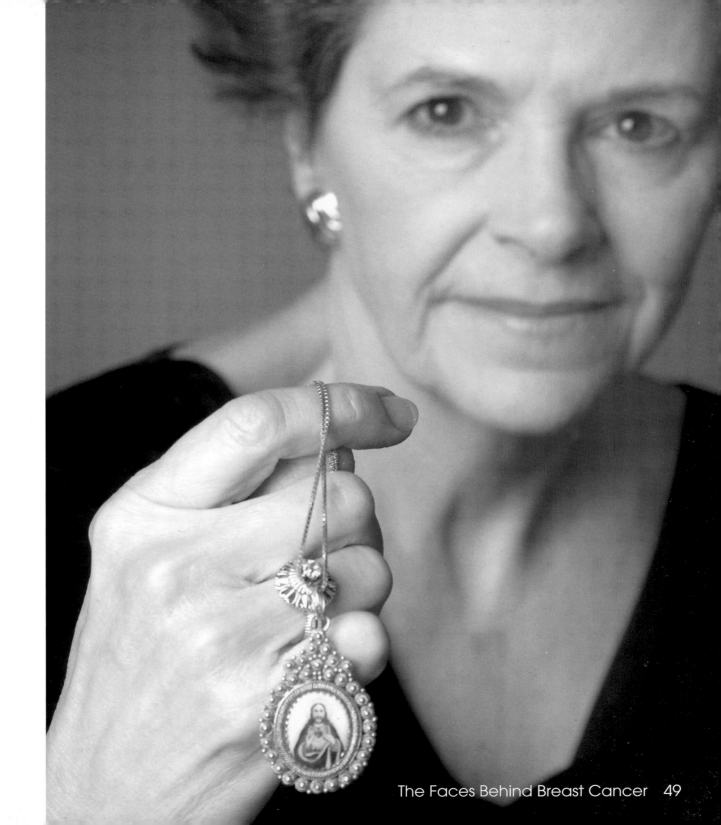

Debra

"I recently celebrated 'year number two' as a breast cancer survivor. As I reflect on the past 24 months, I am different physically, but more profoundly different emotionally. I have released the insignificant and embraced the presence of my faith, family and friends. I am stronger now and gratefully share my journey to encourage my sisters."

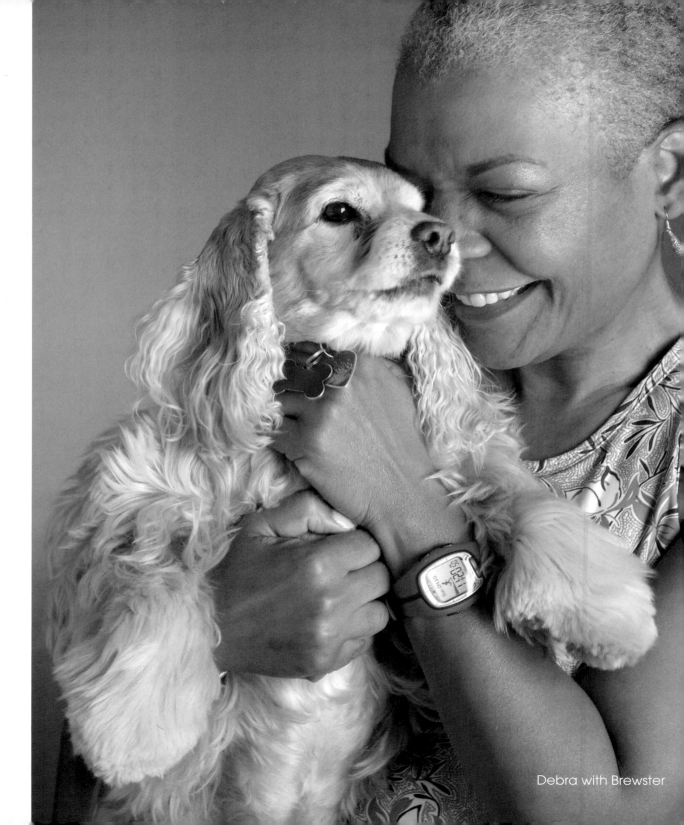

Debra with Brewster

Monique

"My illness brought forth a plethora of emotions. As a result, I have become a more compassionate person. I am more apt to rejoice in someone's triumph as well as cry in their moments of sadness."

Monique & Isabelle

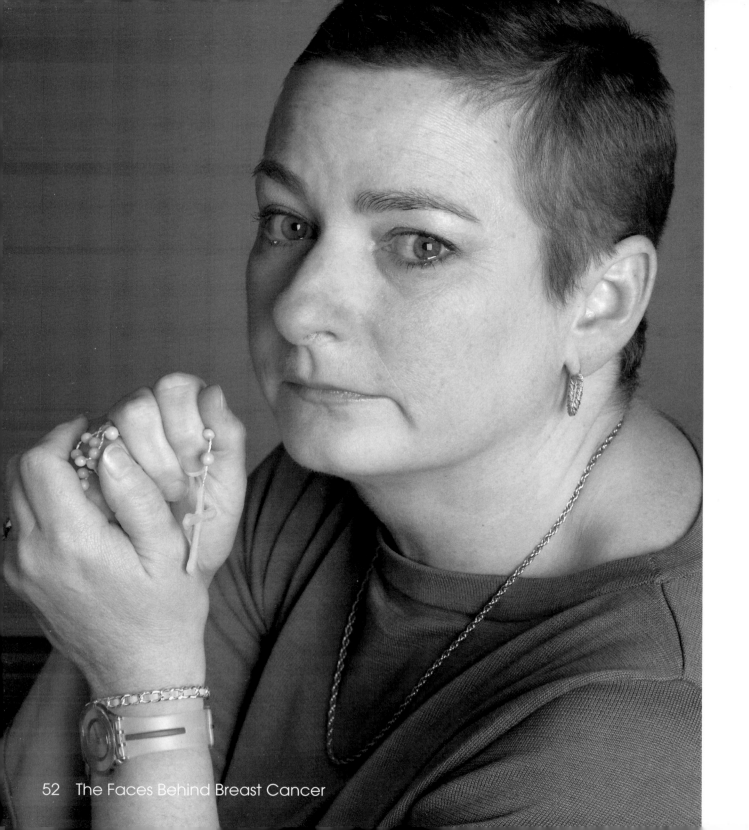

Maike

"This journey has been an inward discovery of my inner strength and God's presence in myself and others."

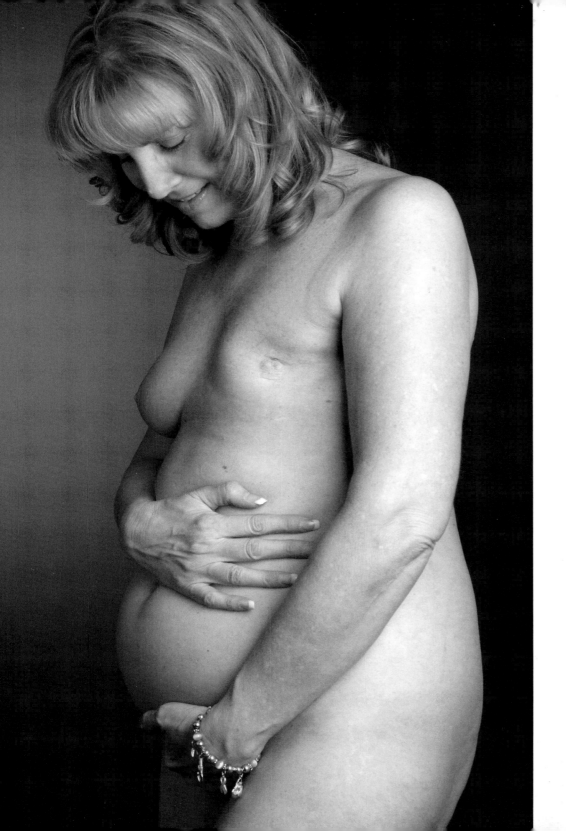

Brenda

"I'm flying high on Life."

Julia

"Breast cancer has made me appreciate my time with my family to the fullest."

Julia & mother, Mrs. Josie

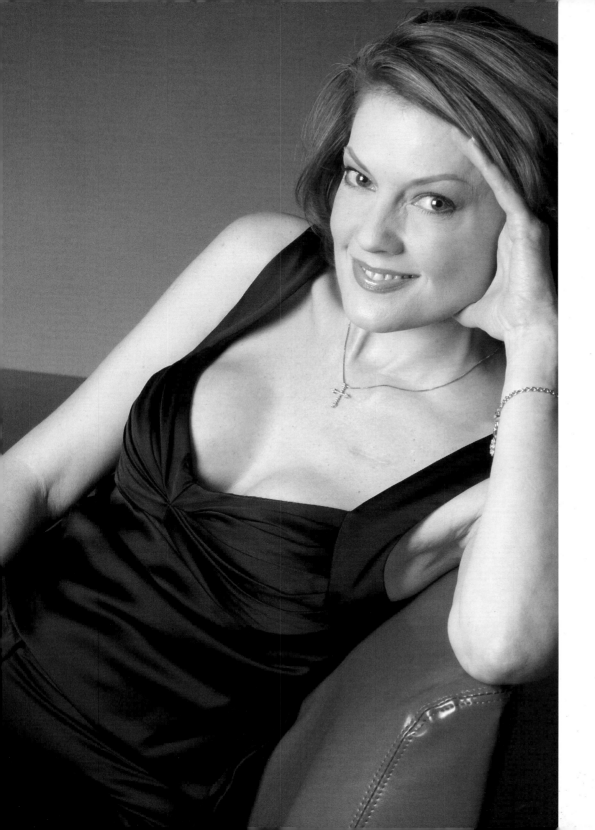

Molly

"I can do all things through Christ who strengthens me.
I can do anything after chemo. As a two-time breast
cancer survivor, I feel that I am able to see things more
clearly and definitely appreciate everything in life–more
so than before my diagnosis."

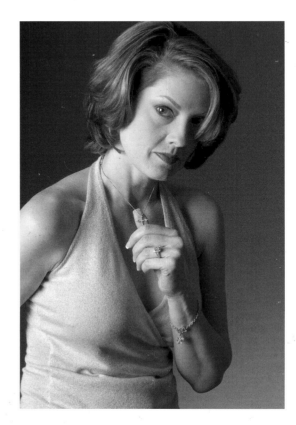

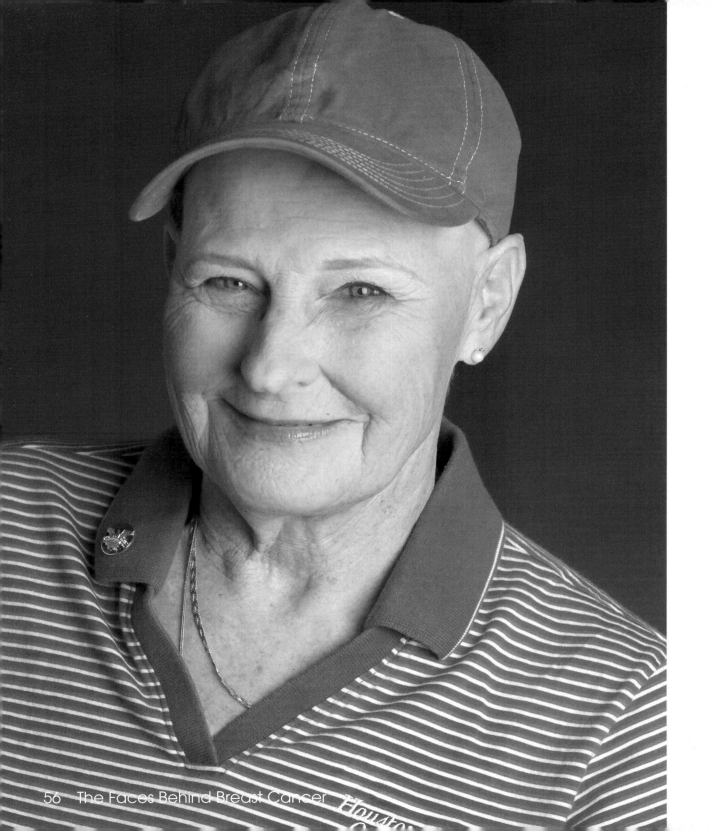

Pat

"Cancer changes your focus. Materialistic pursuits are replaced by concentrating on relationships with family and friends and reaching out to help others. Life is a precious gift from God. Open it daily and laugh more, love more and savor the memories."

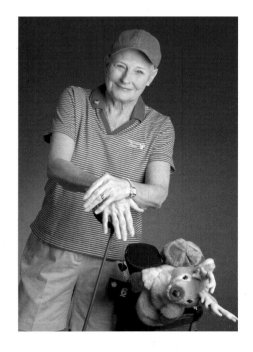

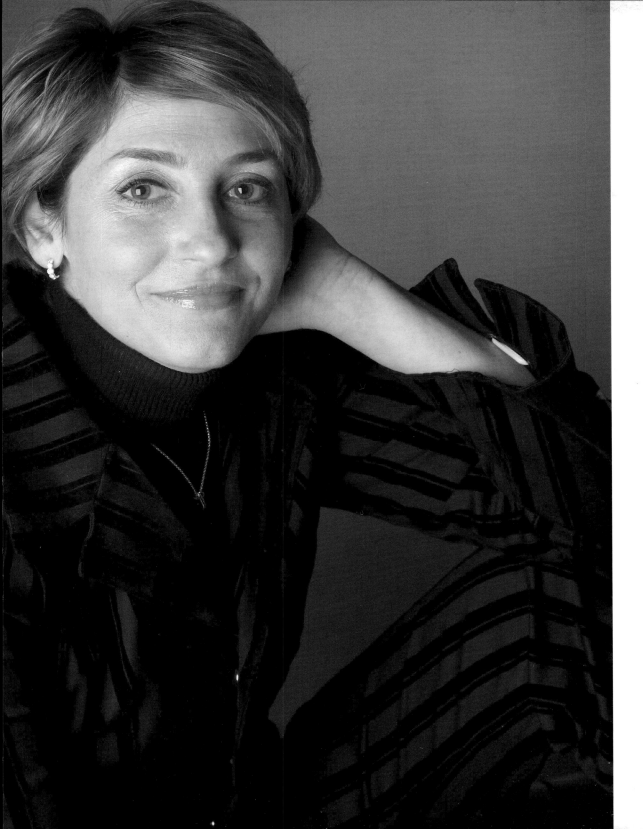

Denise

"We are one hope strong . . . a sentiment that inspired me as I went through treatment, and one that continues to give me hope. Cancer may have knocked me down a few times, but each time I got up, I was stronger and more resilient. I am strong. I am a fighter. I am a survivor."

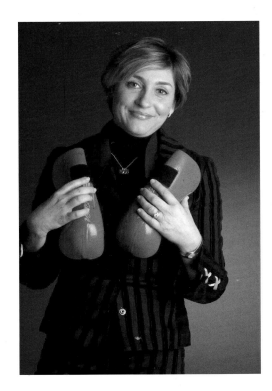

Michelle

"As a physician you are used to taking care of others. During training, and sometimes in practice, you are expected to stay up all night on call for the hospital, and to be on call in the evenings and on weekends. You may think that you have to be invulnerable, but you aren't. You have no control over getting cancer. You have to surrender and accept it. There is no other choice. Those around you are also impacted by your illness. Some can deal with it and some cannot. I was happy to learn that a lot of my relationships were not one-sided. There were people who really cared about me, and I did not even recognize this until I became ill. I learned about gratitude. I learned to better appreciate the goodness and caring of those around me. I began to worry a lot less about superficial things and superficial appearances.

My family prayed for me and patients prayed for me.

I worked as much as I could to keep my mind away

from my illness. Every time I became sick and started

vomiting after chemotherapy, my husband came

running to be with me. He held my shoulders and

wiped off my forehead. He brought me mint tea to

help with the nausea. He was a physician in India, but

gave up his career to take care of me."

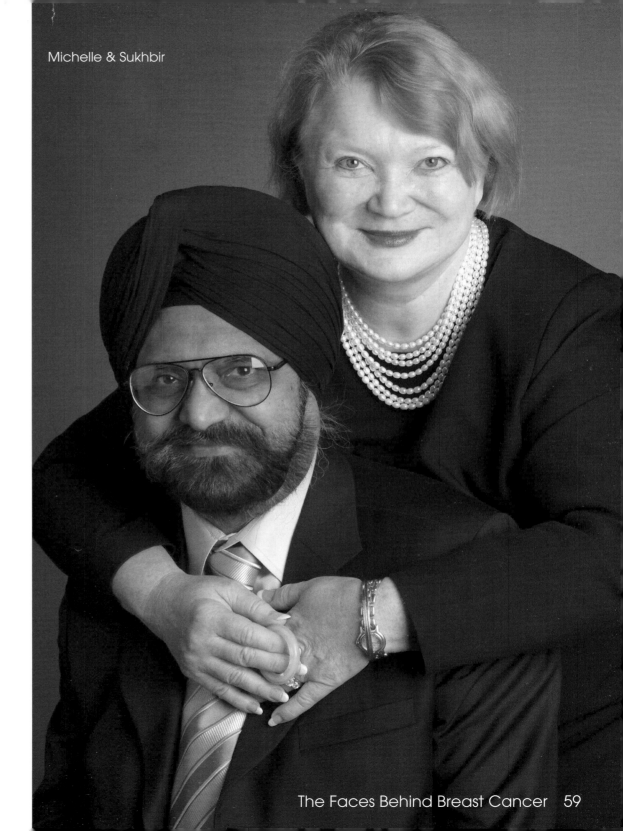

Michelle & Sukhbir

Elizabeth

"As a second-generation survivor whose best friend is also a survivor, breast cancer has affected every aspect of my life. My mother is now terminal, after a nearly 13-year fight with metastatic disease. This disease has affected my family, my marriage, my friendships and my work. We are only human, though, and we are strong. We will persevere and survive, if not in body, then in spirit."

Author's Note: Sadly, Elizabeth's mother passed away on April 11, 2007. She did not live to see her daughter's brave pictorial, but we know she would have been proud.

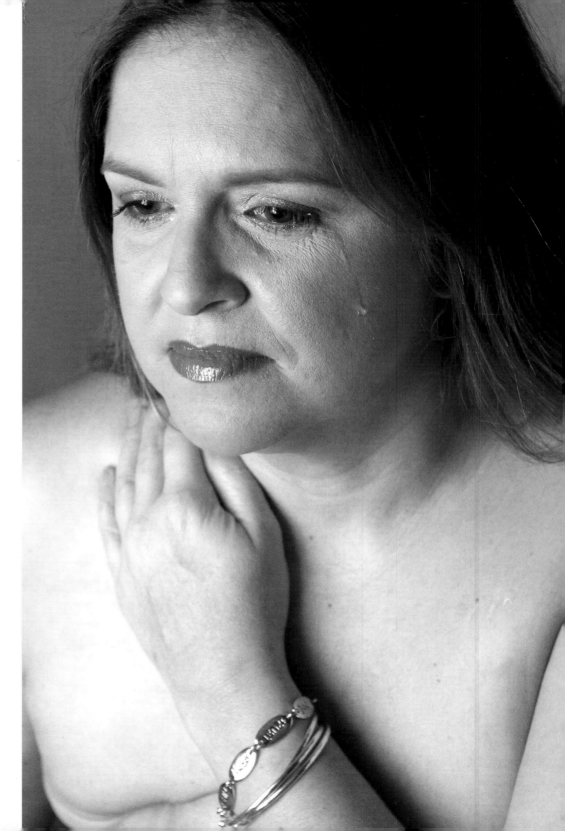

Nancy

"I thought breast cancer would kill me, leaving my young family alone. Instead, the experience brought life and countless freedoms: the freedom to say 'NO,' the freedom to ask for help instead of doing it all, the freedom to honor grief and happiness with my support group sisters, the freedom to evolve spiritually and the freedom to explore nontraditional methods of healing (in stark contrast to my medical career).

Though it sounds crazy, I'm grateful for breast cancer . . . I'm a much better person."

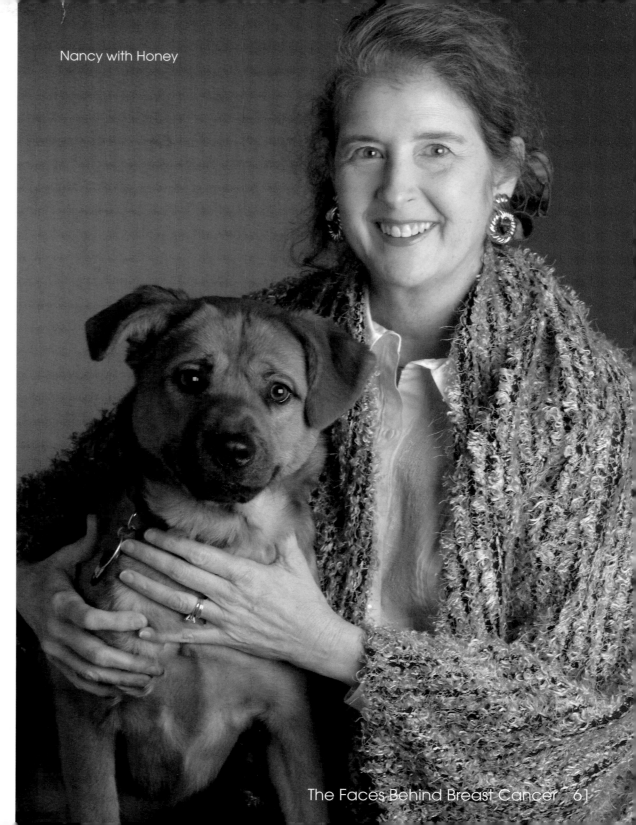

Nancy with Honey

Betsey

"I had a lumpectomy on the 13th of February, 2002. Finding out there was no cancer in my lymph nodes was the best Valentine's present I ever received. And, still now, whether full of joy or sorrow, every day is an incredible gift."

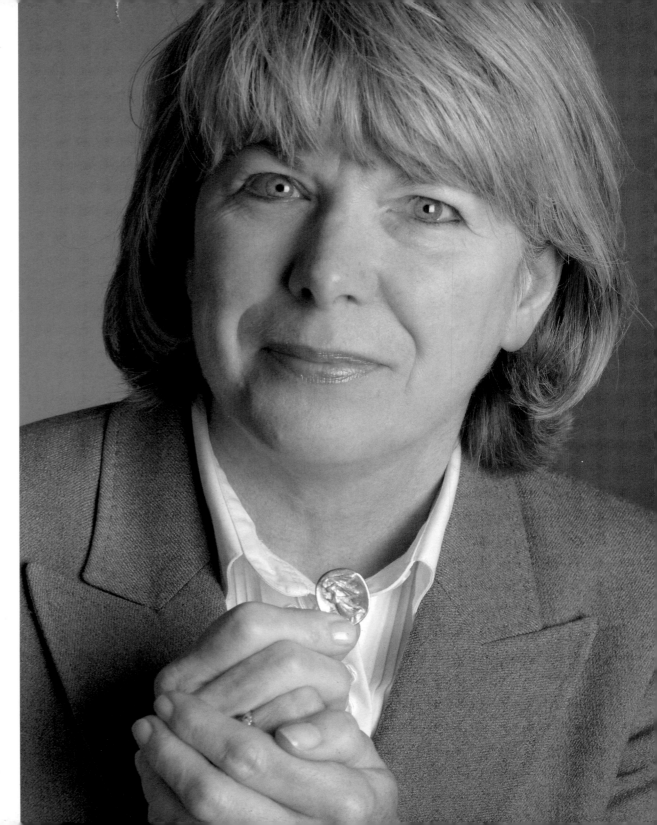

Margaret

"Breast cancer is a way of life for my family. By my mother's example, I learned to teach my daughter awareness. It is the best weapon."

Margaret & daughter Michaela

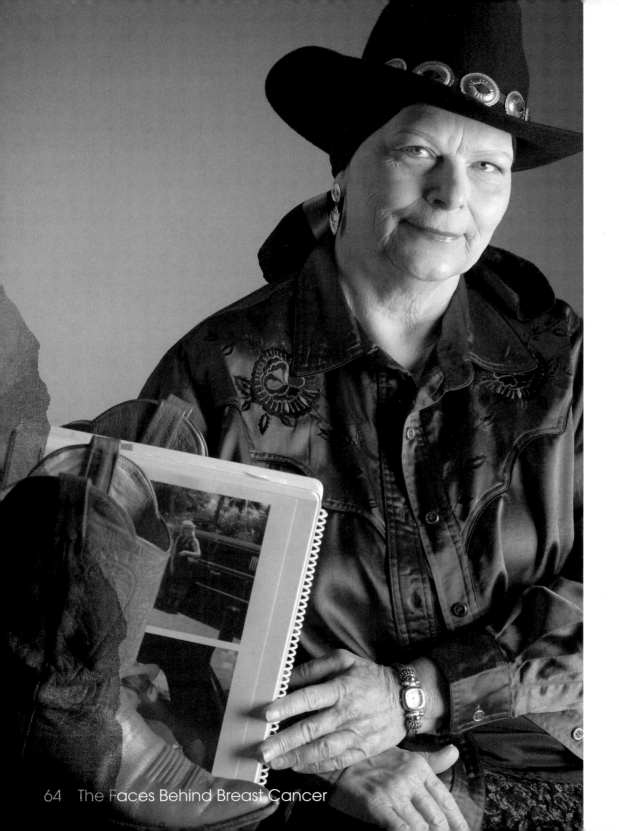

Judy

"Life's a dance: Sometimes you lead, sometimes you follow."

"Until I discovered a lump in my breast in May 2006 and was diagnosed with invasive ductal carcinoma, I had been the nurturer, the family financial and legal advisor, a Houston Livestock Show & Rodeo Committee volunteer, a Houston Volunteer Lawyer monthly legal aid clinic volunteer, a Hobby Center volunteer, a paralegal and a dance instructor. I was a leader. In my time of need, my family and friends became my guardian angels and led me to realize how important I was to everyone else, giving me a positive attitude and a will to survive. As soon as I complete my aggressive 15-month treatment plan, I shall lead and dance again!"

Wendy

"Cancer has given me a greater appreciation of my life and for all of those I love. It has also given me a greater commitment to enjoy each day to its fullest. As a survivor, I try to reach out and help as many other women going through their journey with cancer as I can."

Wendy & Lewis

Emily

"I have learned that the most important thing in life is the journey, not the destination . . . and that true happiness comes from within a person. God blessed me with such special children, friends and family who helped me find the strength and courage that have always been there. With His grace we will continue wherever the road takes us, and I look forward to every day."

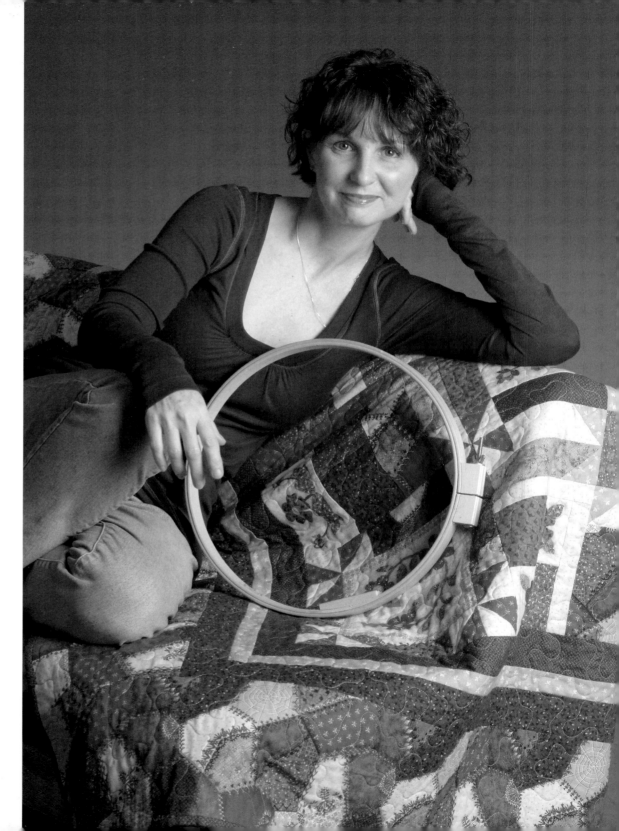

Allen

"This experience has allowed me to step outside my own experience and be an inspiration to others."

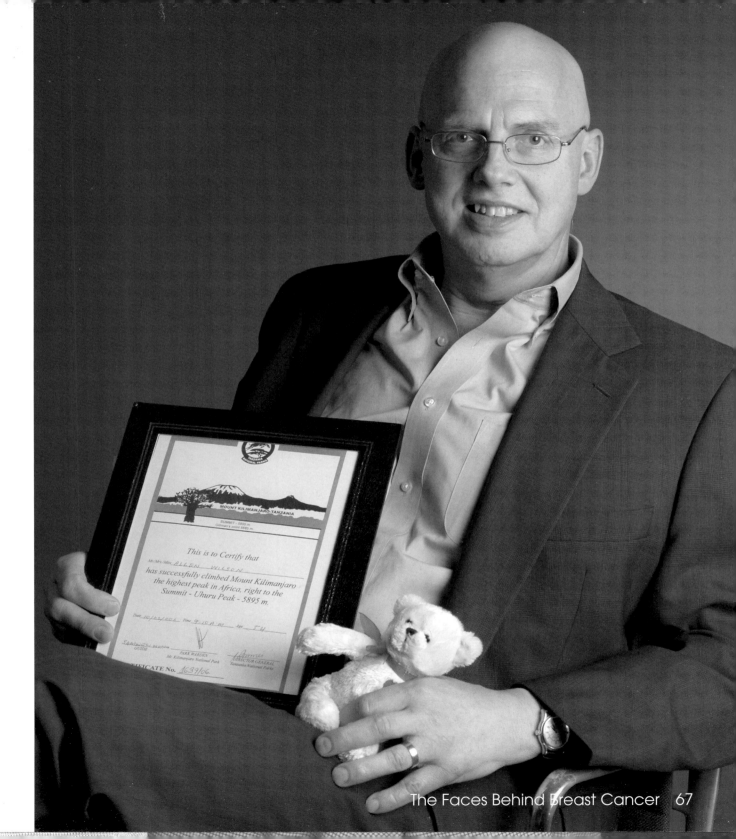

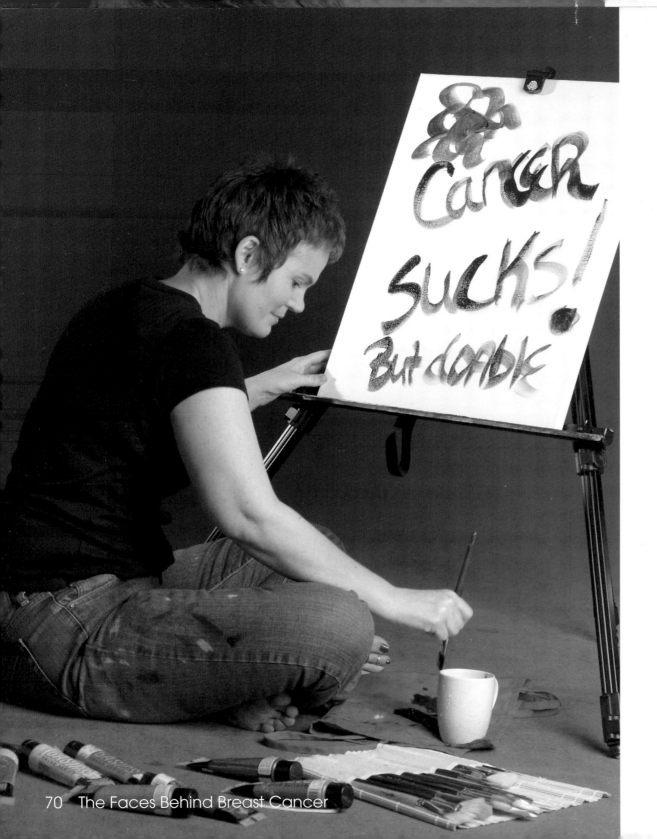

Beverly

"Breast cancer has opened my eyes to a new me and a new world. I found I am a much stronger person once I saw the courage inside."

Allen

"This experience has allowed me to step outside my own experience and be an inspiration to others."

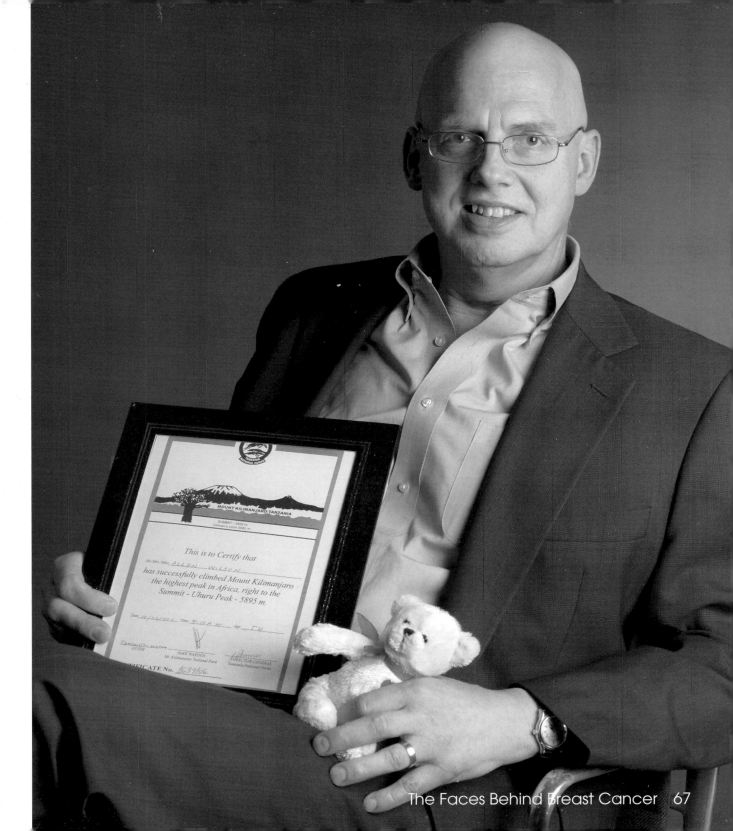

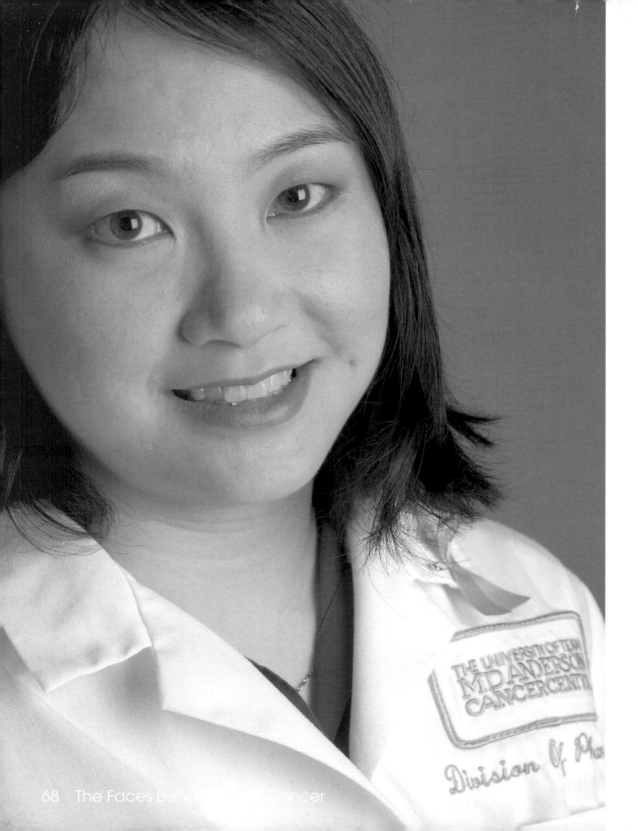

Victoria

"More or less, breast cancer has changed my life.

I fear less, worry less, hate less, and love more,

appreciate more, laugh more and live more."

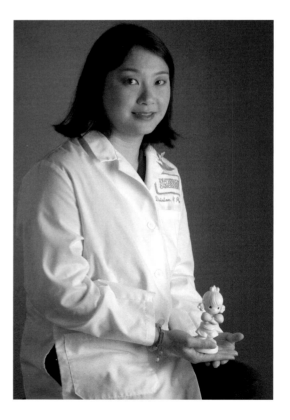

Flo

"I would say that I could not have been able to get through my cancer treatment without Jesus Christ, my wonderful and loving husband Jim and the support of friends. Also, new friends I have met along this road are a gift and blessing to me."

Flo & Jim

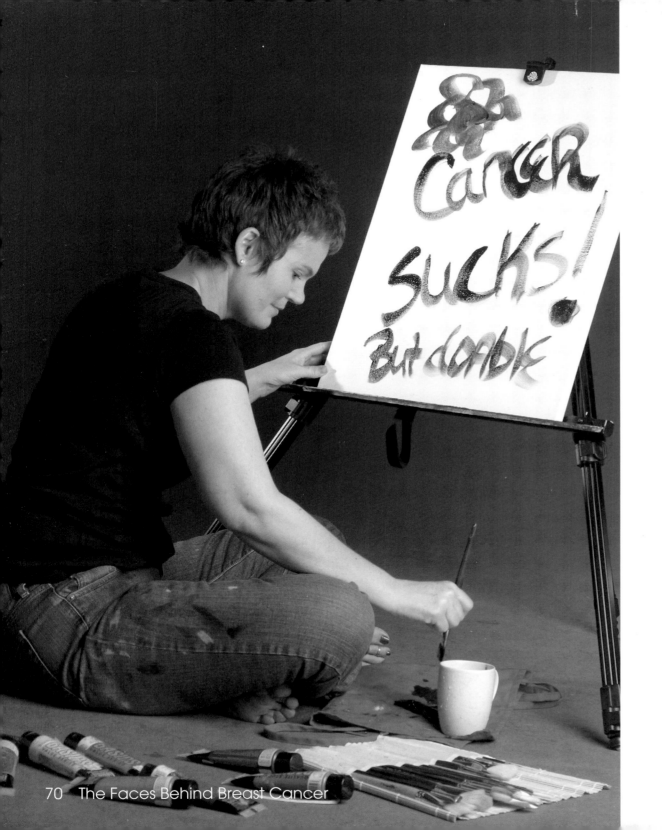

Cancer
SUCKS!
But doable

Beverly

"Breast cancer has opened my eyes to a new me and a new world. I found I am a much stronger person once I saw the courage inside."

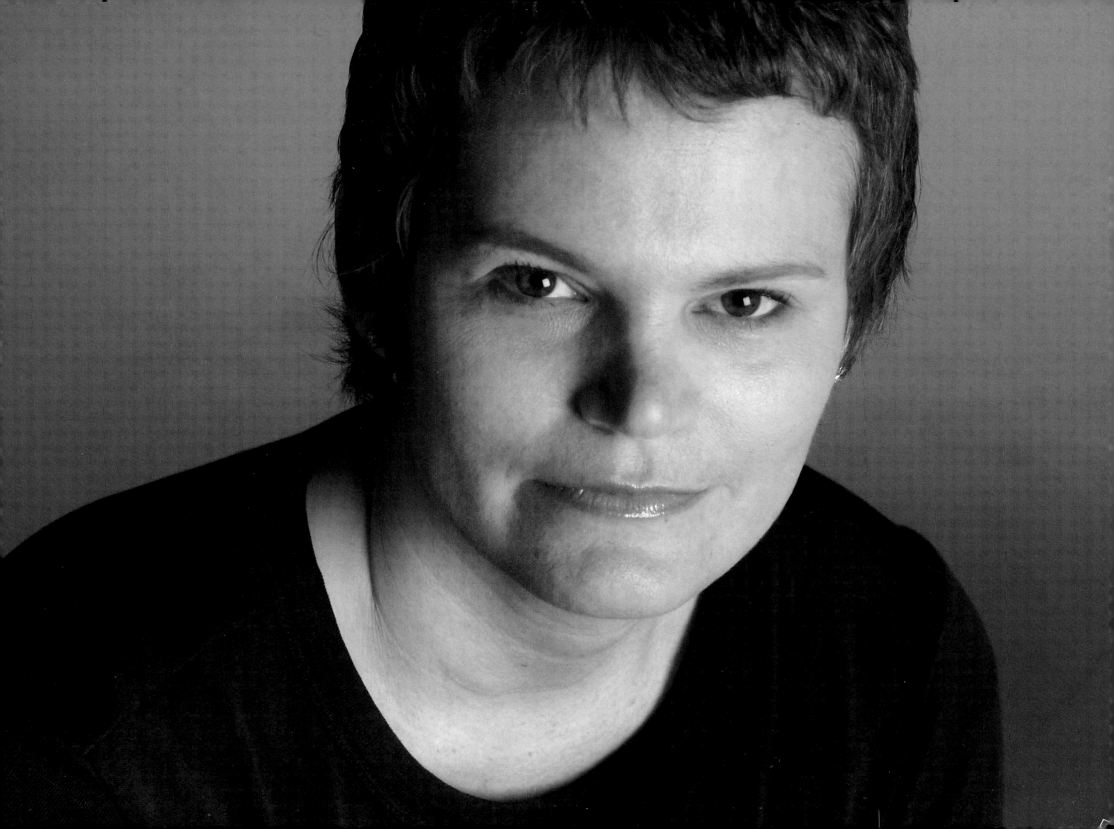

Mary

"I realized that life is too short and we need to live every day as if it is our last. Without the Lord to lean on, I could not have made it through my breast cancer. Psalm 144 was my scripture. My song was "If You Want Me To" by Ginny Owens, AND, most of all, thank you to my friends and ex-husband that were there for me. I am now 8 years out."

Marsha

"Carpe diem. There is an old Indian saying: 'When you were born, you cried and the world rejoiced. Live your life in such a manner that when you die, the world cries and you rejoice.'"

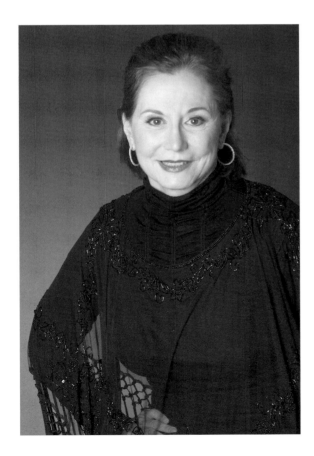

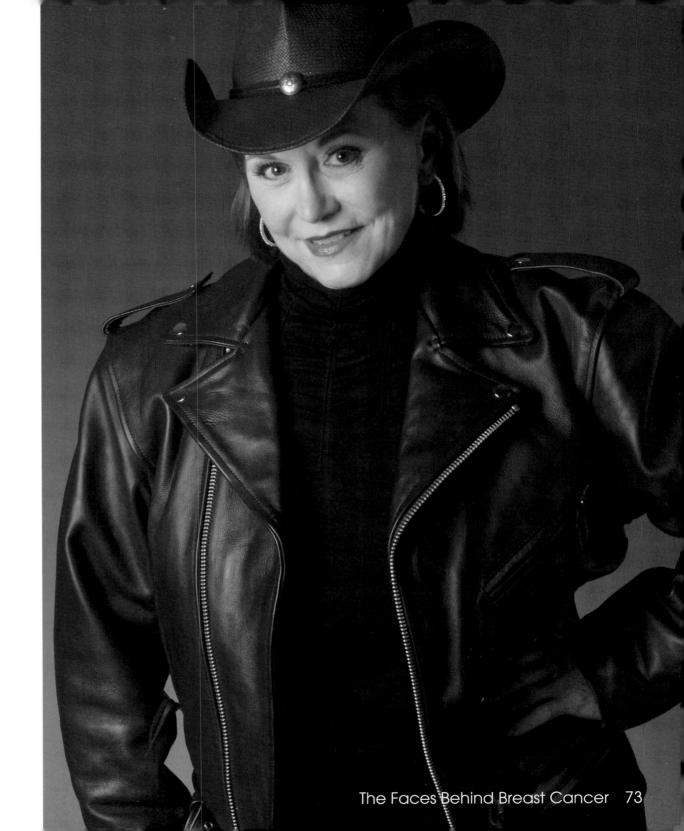

Rosemary

"My breast cancer experience changed my priorities. It taught me what is really important in life. It strengthened my relationship with my husband, my primary caregiver and number one supporter."

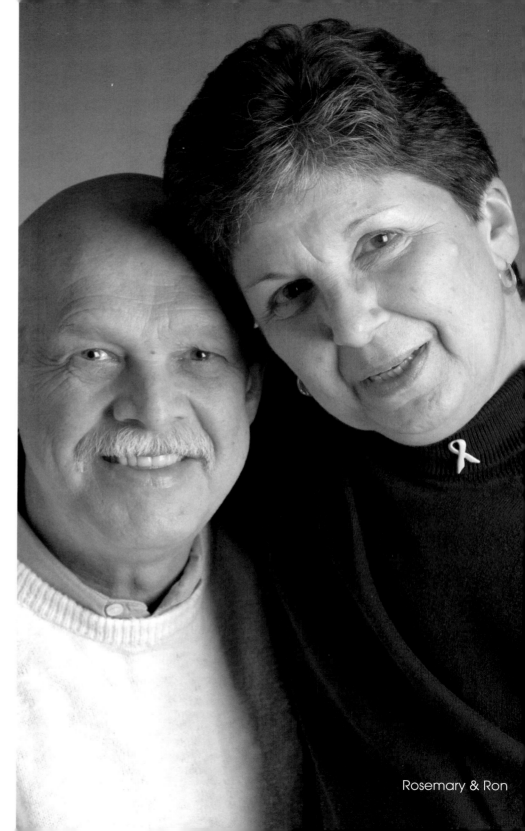

Rosemary & Ron

Claudine

"Life is precious; don't take it for granted. To whom much is given, much is required. More important, through all things trust and depend on God."

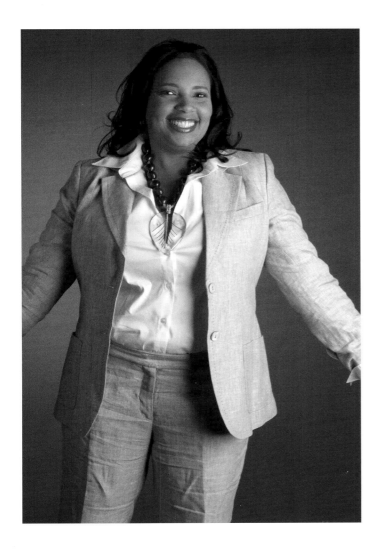

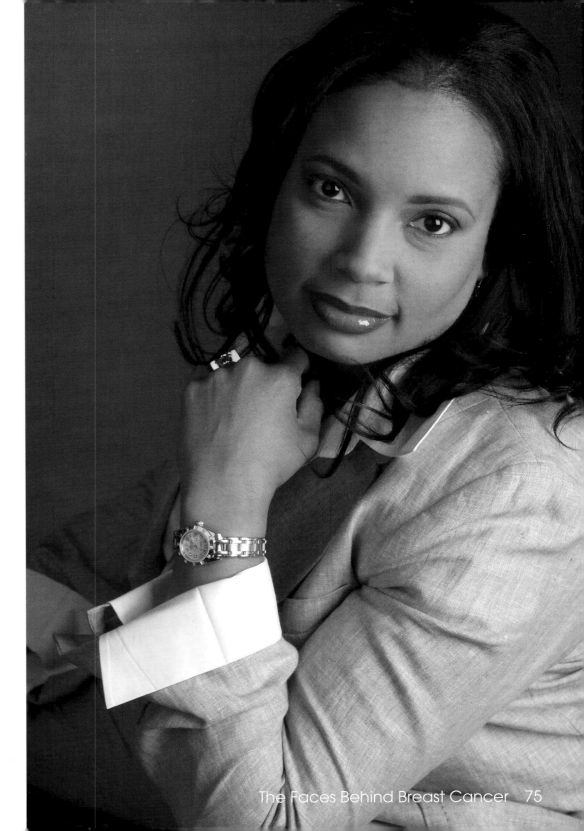

Laura

"For me, my cancer has made me see the grass greener, the sky bluer and my children's faces more precious! I live each day with the end in mind."

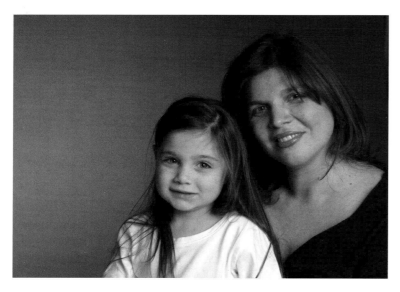

Laura with daughter Amelia & friend Suzanne

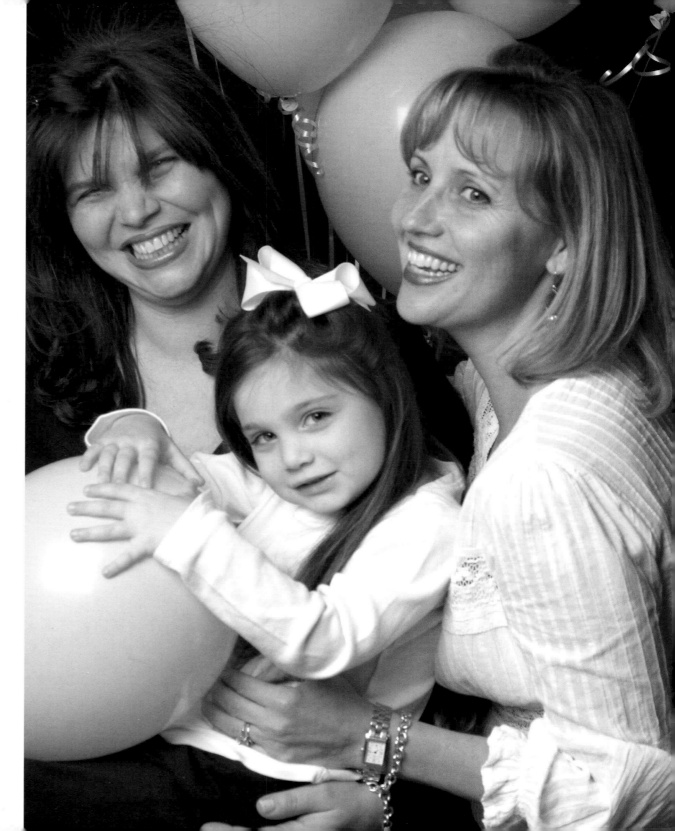

Chris

"Having cancer has taught me that I can handle whatever life tosses my way. I am more confident and peaceful, and better able to let go of things that don't matter, while focusing on the things that do. I believe in my strength, and I have learned how to use it to live well. I wear a medallion inscribed with the date of the end of my treatment: October 3, 2006."

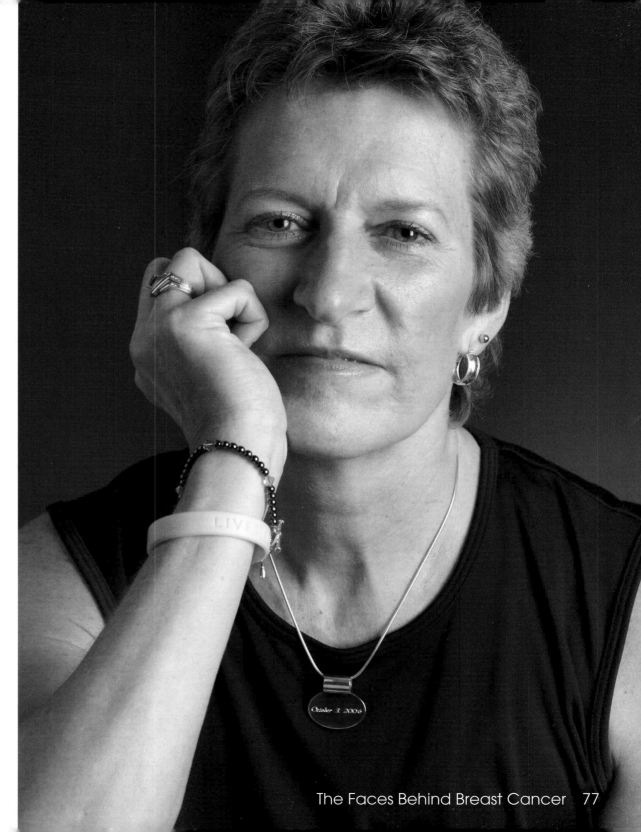

Karissa

"I was diagnosed four months after I was married. It threw us from being newlyweds into an uncertain future. I quickly learned what was important and what was not important in life. I think everything happens for a reason. I now believe my reason was to help educate young women about breast cancer."

Donna

"Live for the moment and enjoy your family and

friends. Dance as if no one is watching."

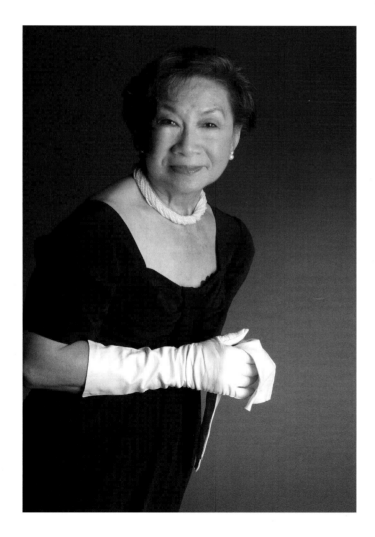

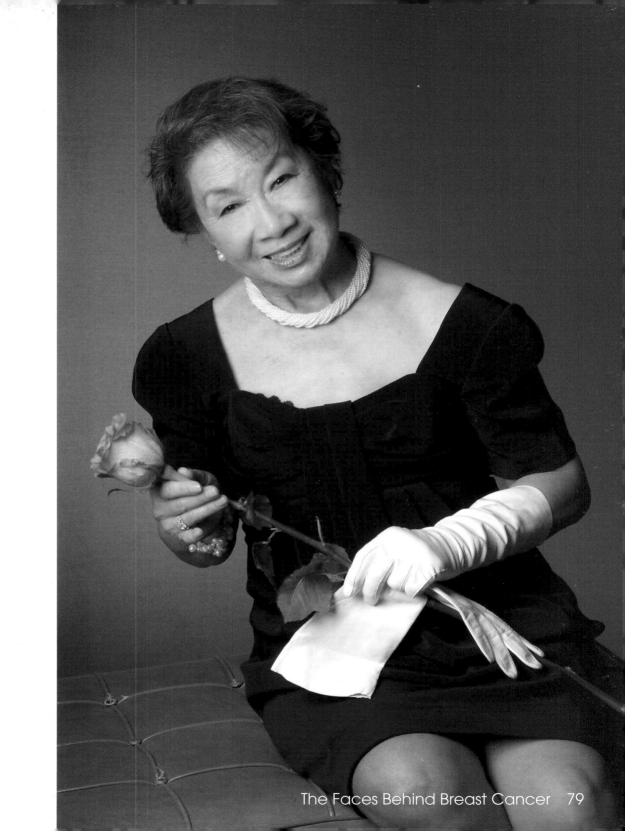

Doug

"I didn't think breast cancer was a disease that men could get. My initial embarrassment and inclination to keep it secret gave way to an admission that I needed help from others—and not just the doctors. I was reminded that what I couldn't manage alone, together we could deal with. There is great power in a crisis shared. I am here now to pass along the help that was given to me so generously."

Jeannie

"My life is better, richer and deeper!! Besides my faith in Christ, my husband's love, humor and encouragement were truly the backbone that kept me going during treatment, and he continues to lift me up each day!

Through breast cancer, God has also given me a heart for and a ministry to those who are hurting and an appreciation for every day He allows me to serve Him!"

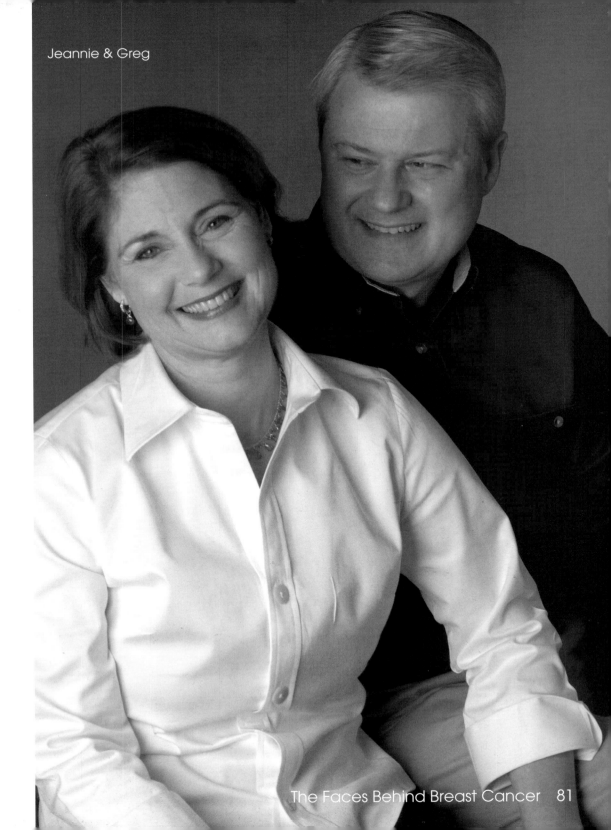

Jeannie & Greg

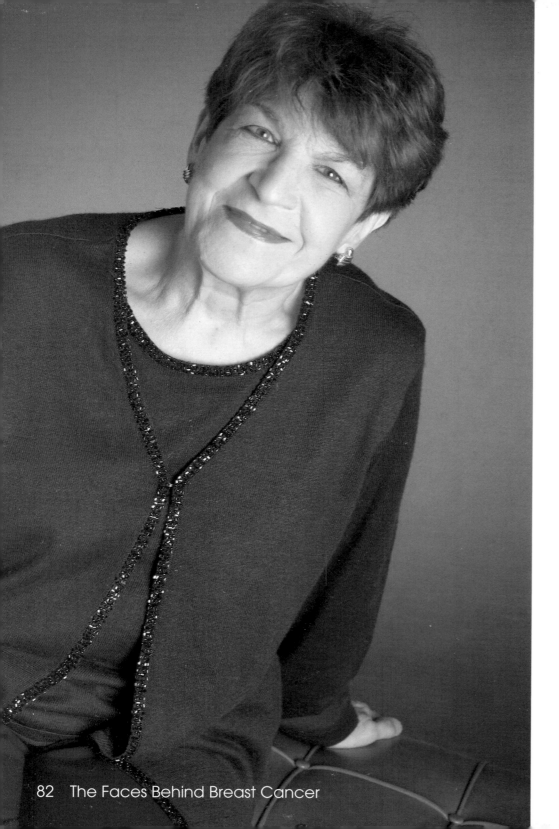

Josie M.

"Cancer awakened my heart and opened my eyes to the world around me. I saw that I had much for which to be grateful. The joy of my Lord continues to be my strength."

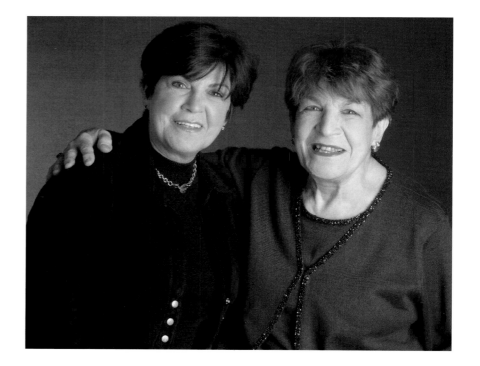

Josie M. with sister Catherine, daughter Margaret, niece Lisa

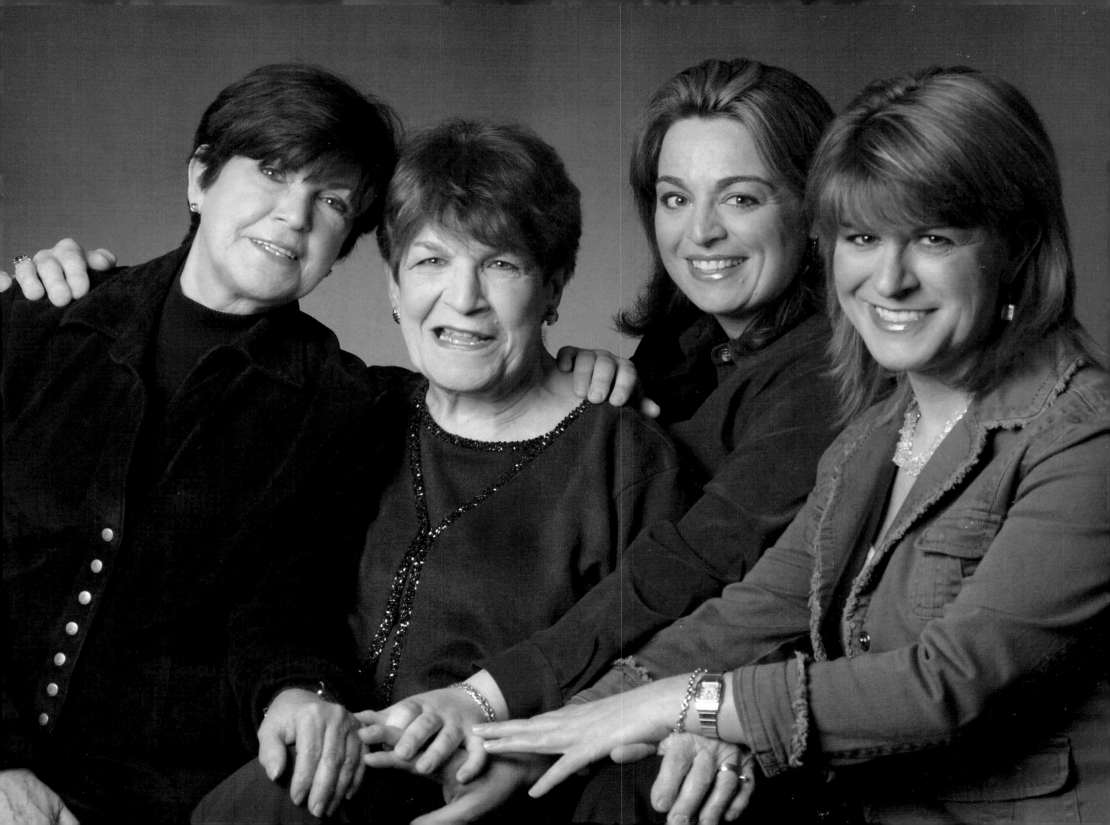

Susan

"I've learned to say NO and mean it (mostly anyway). I've learned to take it one day at a time and sometimes one step at a time when things are overwhelming. And, I've learned to build sand castles even when the tide is coming in."

Sonia

"The experience of cancer treatments has

added a new dimension to my life, as well as

expanded my current lifestyle to new horizons

I never knew existed."

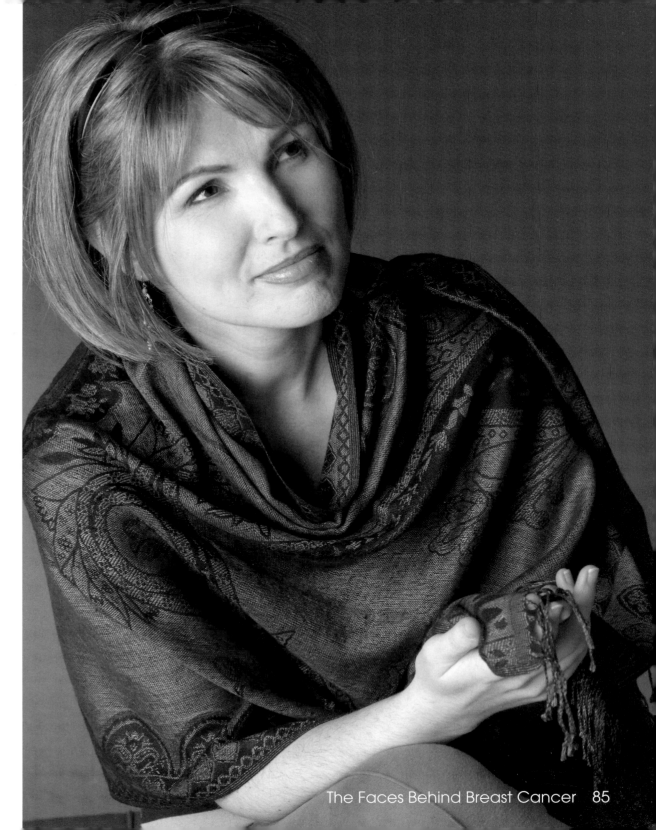

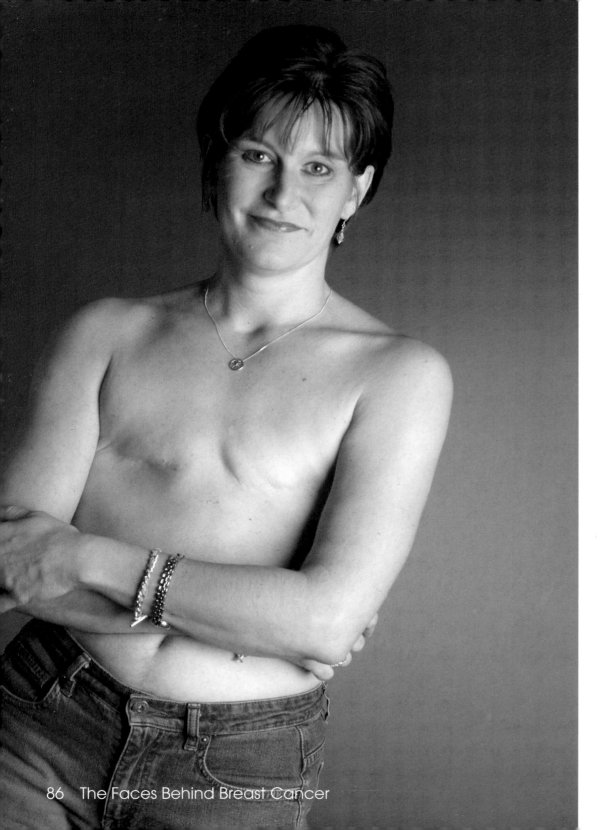

Susan

"Attitude will help get you through anything. It's 90 percent. Whatever else you do is 10 percent. Once a complete control fanatic, I've realized through my breast cancer battle not to sweat the small stuff! God only gives you what you can handle, although you may not agree with Him. He will get you through."

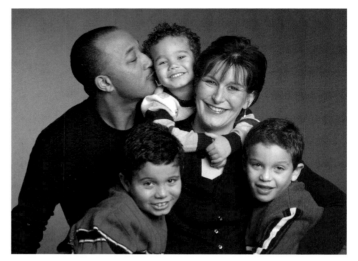

Susan with husband Elliott & sons Elliott III, William & Jonathan

Michelle

"When I returned to work full time, I met with a colleague with whom I had limited interaction the previous (and my first) year. She took a moment before I left her office to share with me how she had watched me from afar as I progressed through my chemotherapy, surgeries and radiation. She admired my courage to continue working and to be out in public with my hats and, toward the end, with just a faint carpet of hair. Her words of admiration were a shock to me. I never once thought of myself in that way; I was only trying my best to still be a part of life."

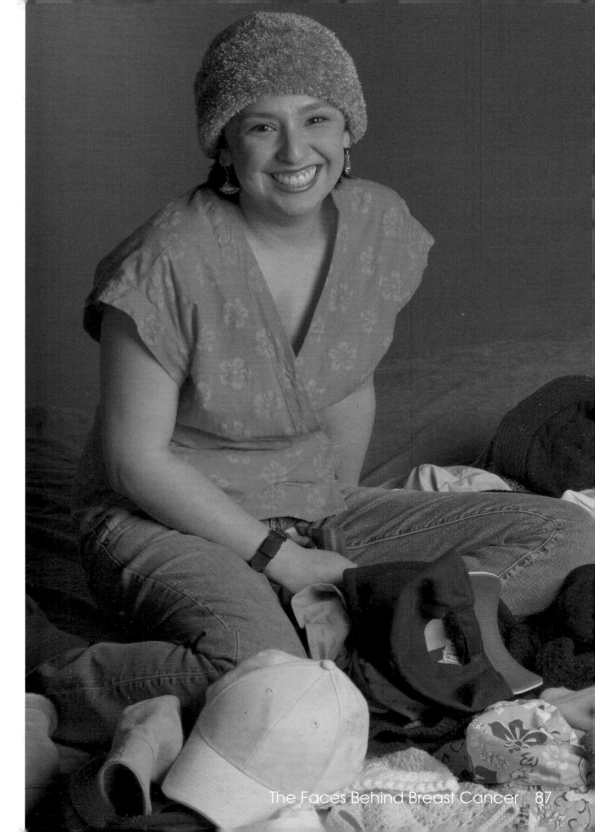

Julia

"Breast cancer has given me a purpose in life: to inform, to educate, to support and to inspire others through their cancer journey. I hope that my experiences will inspire others to keep going."

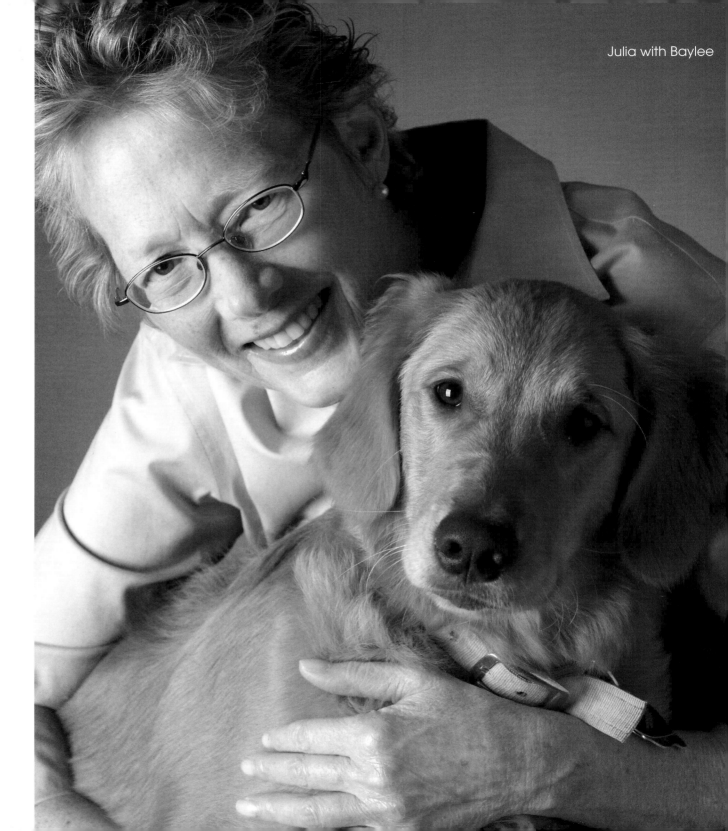

Julia with Baylee

Janet

"Now that I am five years out, survivorship has taken on a much deeper meaning."

Juli & daughter Jessica

Juli

"Seeing my daughter go through a brain tumor gave me the strength I needed one year later to get through my breast cancer diagnosis. I would say cancer has made me less afraid of life, like flying and all sorts of things."

Author's Note: Sadly, Juli's courageous battle ended in May 2007. We hope her family will find comfort and solace through the legacy of this pictorial, knowing she remains a source of inspiration to everyone who sees it. She will be missed but never forgotten.

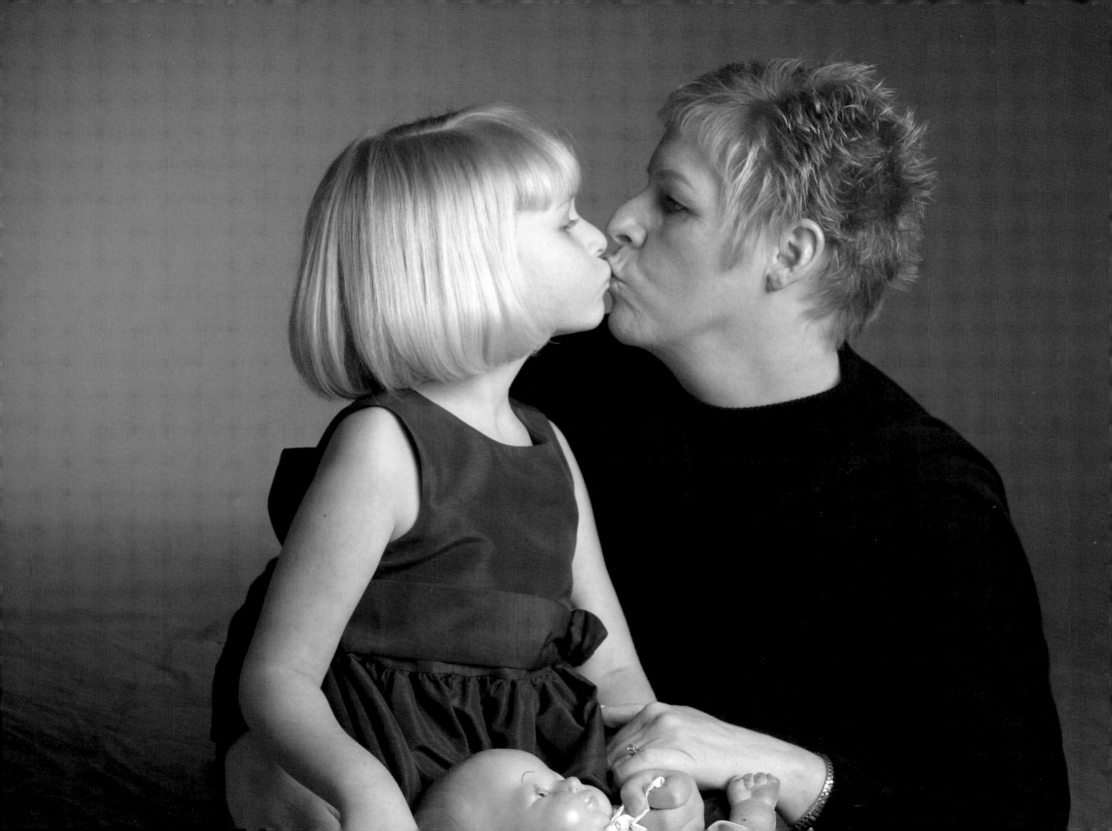

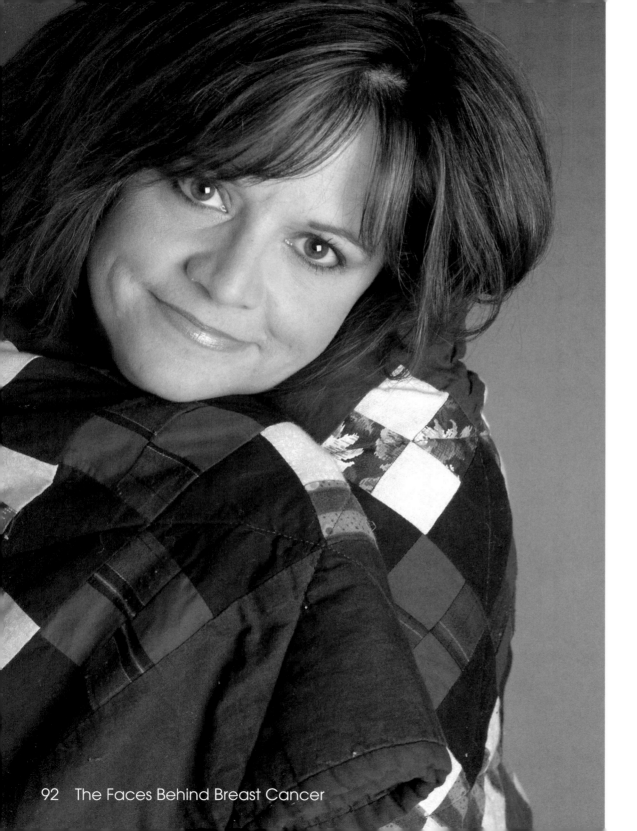

Sara

"Since my diagnosis and treatment, I have learned that I am blessed by His grace. I have all the strength and courage I need to survive, and it is all because of His grace."

Physicians & Staff

Oncology

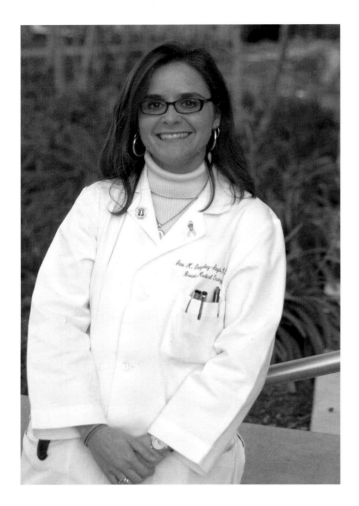

Ana Maria Gonzalez-Angulo, M.D.

Assistant Professor of Breast Medical Oncology

M. D. Anderson Cancer Center

Twenty-five years ago I had my first encounter with cancer. Within a year I lost someone I loved, but was inspired by his brother who assumed the difficult task of being both family and physician.

My aunt was 35 when she died, and I promised myself I would do something to help others who are going down the same path.

Here I am today, listening to the laughter of beautiful women with sparkling, bald heads. Their laughter is infectious, touching everyone with a warm feeling. They are anxious, but they have hope.

In particular, I met a woman three years ago who had been diagnosed with breast cancer that had unfortunately spread to her brain. The doctors had all told her the same thing: "You have six months, put your affairs in order." She burst into my life, crying, begging for hope. "I have a son I want to see graduate. I need enough time," she said to me.

I knew the statistics were grim. I knew that what the other physicians had told her was true. I looked at her and said, "I can't promise you anything, but I will do everything I can to help you."

Three years down the road, she is still here and keeps her appointments without fail. She continues chemotherapy to keep the disease under control, and is doing well, having beaten all odds. She attended her son's high school graduation, and he will soon be out of college. When I see her, I think back and see a smile from above. I remember to live each day to the fullest as my patients do.

Radiation Oncology

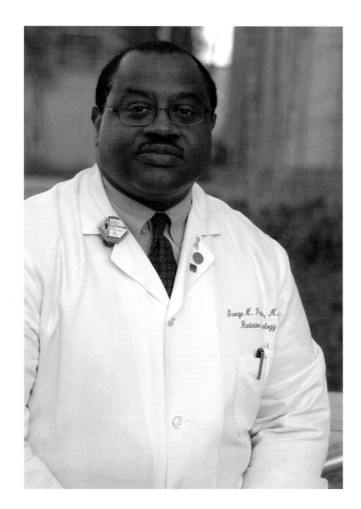

George H. Perkins, M.D.
Associate Professor of Radiation Oncology
M. D. Anderson Cancer Center

"You know, Dr. Perkins, cancer changes you." These words uttered by a recent patient resonated with me. As a radiation oncologist with expertise in breast disease and outcomes, I know the way cancer changes the body, and I know the way that our treatments change the cancer. My patients afford me the privilege of learning how our treatments change them and how cancer changes the individual. I am grateful for the patients who share their families, dreams and fears with me. I honor the trust that they give me to develop a treatment plan best suited for the amelioration of their disease. When I prescribe radiation to tumors, I commit to being responsive to the whole patient: medically, spiritually and emotionally.

Why? It is because cancer changes you. One of the reasons I specialize in oncology is my personal experience with cancer in my family. At times bravery evolves from fear, joy blooms amid despair, hope springs from sorrow and grace dances around destitution. At other times, all of the nouns reverse. "Cancer changes you, yet it does not have to define you. Sometimes you feel like you are withstanding enormous pressure." Well, in my experience with patients at M. D. Anderson, pressure makes diamonds! I thank God for the opportunity to assist as a "jeweler."

Surgical Oncology

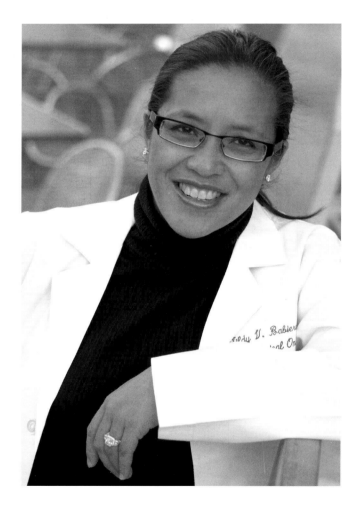

Gildy Babiera, M.D.
Assistant Professor of Surgical Oncology
M. D. Anderson Cancer Center

Early in my breast surgical oncology career, I treated a 30-year-old indigent patient who would travel four hours on a bus from West Texas to come to M. D. Anderson Cancer Center for her breast cancer care. God knows what she had to do to get to the bus terminal. She had no family in Houston, or for that matter, at home in West Texas. I performed her surgery, which required an overnight stay. She recovered in a motel in Houston, alone, except for the visiting nurse who came to see her once every day. She left on a bus to return to West Texas after spending three days alone.

During her treatment, never once did I hear her complain or expect more than what we could give. To this day, I will always remember her small, frail body and her innocent eyes, trusting that I would do the best for her and hoping for a cure.

As I look back, I was blessed to be able to have met someone with such courage and dignity. She taught me that every person is an individual, and that cancer care not only includes the medical and surgical treatments we offer, but that it also includes listening to our patients and finding out who they are and what is important to them. I thank her and all of my patients for the privilege of allowing me to be part of their lives and for teaching me many of life's valuable lessons: Do not take for granted the life that we live and cherish each and every moment.

Reconstructive Surgery

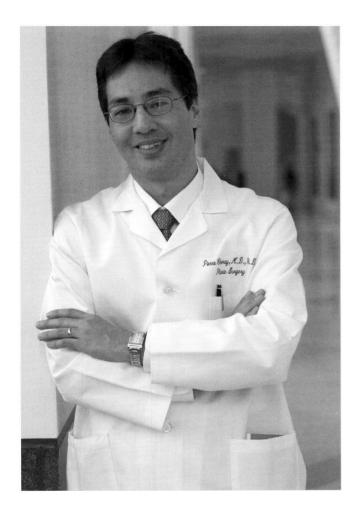

Pierre Chevray, M.D., Ph. D.
Associate Professor of Plastic Surgery
M. D. Anderson Cancer Center

Breast reconstruction is a delicate balance of reconstructive and cosmetic surgery. I am a plastic and reconstructive surgeon who practices this art and science.

Most patients come to me with uncertainty, concerns and fears. Many have just recently found out that they have breast cancer. Others have already been through months of chemotherapy, radiation treatments and surgery. Some patients have researched breast reconstruction and know exactly what they want. However, most patients have very little idea what a reconstructed breast will be like. They need careful explanation of the types of breast reconstruction available to them and an honest discussion of what to expect.

Sometimes patients are more comfortable seeing photographic examples of breast reconstructions or speaking to others who have had breast reconstruction surgery. Ultimately, it is the patient's decision as to when and what type of breast reconstruction to have.

Breast reconstructive surgery is not perfect, and the realistic goal is to have every patient appear normal and symmetric in clothing. The larger goal is to restore a patient's self-esteem and positive-body image, and allow her to return to her life and forget she ever had breast cancer. My best days are ones when a patient gives me a hug and sincere thanks for making her feel whole again, or when she tells me she has returned to her daily routine and forgotten that she had a mastectomy and breast reconstruction. I always have to suppress a smile when I examine a patient and notice a tan line on her chest that indicates she has been wearing a bathing suit after her breast reconstruction.

The importance of breast reconstruction has been acknowledged in the United States by The Women's Health and Cancer Rights Act of 1998. This is a federal law that requires health insurance companies to cover breast reconstruction, including surgery on the opposite breast to improve symmetry.

Breast & Surgical Pathology

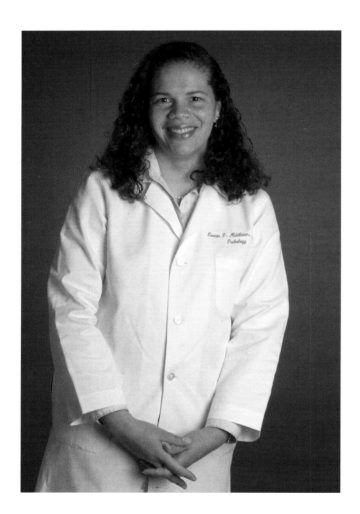

Lavinia Middleton, M.D.
Associate Professor of Pathology
M. D. Anderson Cancer Center

I am a diagnostic surgical pathologist. My primary responsibility is to render timely and accurate diagnoses to aid the oncologist in designing an individualized treatment plan.

By evaluating specimens obtained from patients at the time of surgery, I am able to identify factors that will predict response to therapy.

I have a tremendous amount of job satisfaction because I am able to communicate my observations to the clinician and help formulate a treatment plan. I diagnose cancer every day, sometimes every hour of the day, but it never becomes routine. I am frequently saddened when I make the diagnosis of breast carcinoma and often wonder how the news is going to affect the patient and his or her family.

Although I rarely get the opportunity to communicate directly with the patient, I am a tenacious patient advocate, working with the surgeon and radiologist to achieve negative margins intra-operatively and advising the oncologist on the aggressiveness of a patient's tumor.

I thoroughly enjoy other aspects of my profession, like teaching trainees who rotate through our department and doing clinical-based research.

I am fortunate to work closely with a skilled multidisciplinary team of oncologists dedicated to treating breast cancer. I am blessed to work alongside my husband, Dr. George Perkins, an exemplary radiation oncologist who shares a similar commitment to delivering excellent patient care.

Breast Center Staff

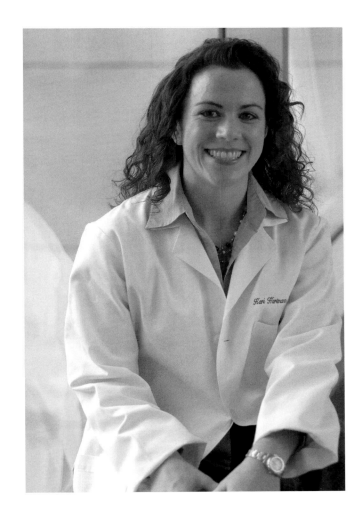

Kari Hartmann
Physician Assistant, Surgical Oncology
M. D. Anderson Cancer Center

Working with breast cancer patients has changed my life. I am continuously impressed by the courage and faith that they show in the midst of a devastating diagnosis. Months of treatment can rob them of their appetite, hair and energy, but they often tell me they're doing great and have no complaints!

I find myself thinking about this positive outlook when things in my life do not go the way I had planned. Attitude really makes a huge difference in the quality of our lives. We have a choice to accept our circumstances and then take charge of those things over which we have control. After that, it is up to us to slow down and appreciate every moment as a gift. I make an effort to take notice of the beauty around me every day and to really be thankful for my health.

My patients express such gratitude for simple things: loving friends and family, an understanding employer, the care they receive during treatment. By following my patients' examples, I am living and loving life in the *present*.

Breast Center Staff

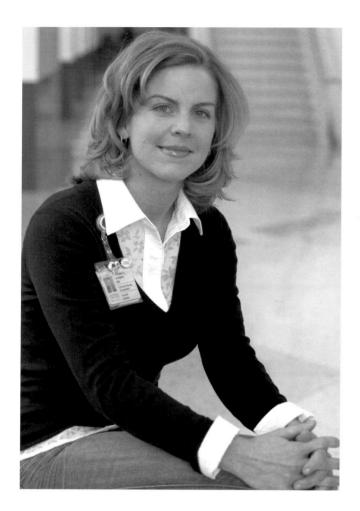

Theresa Johnson, R.N.
Outpatient Clinical Nurse, Breast Center
M. D. Anderson Cancer Center

I always knew that becoming a nurse was my calling in life. I can remember as a child running over to help whenever someone was hurt or not feeling well. The gratification that I would feel when I could make someone better, whether it was emotionally or physically, was so rewarding, and I knew that was my purpose in this world.

Fast forward to here and now. I have been with M. D. Anderson for seven years and am very proud to be a part of such a wonderful hospital. This institution is so sophisticated and so advanced in its medical treatment that it is almost breathtaking. Yet, it retains that warm southern hospitality as if you were being cared for by your own family. The clinic is full of brilliant, caring nurses who shine each and every day. Many patients inform me that M. D. Anderson picks only the best, because we have the most outstanding nursing care they could ask for.

On a daily basis, we care for women "fighting the beast," and knowing that we can help them in any way, whether small or large, is personally fulfilling to me. I cannot dream of doing anything else. The strength of these women will move you and pull at your heart in a way that you could never imagine. They are my inspiration and even though I know I am helping them through their difficult times, they have no idea how much they help me. I am proud to be a part of "Making Cancer History®."

Plastic Surgery Staff

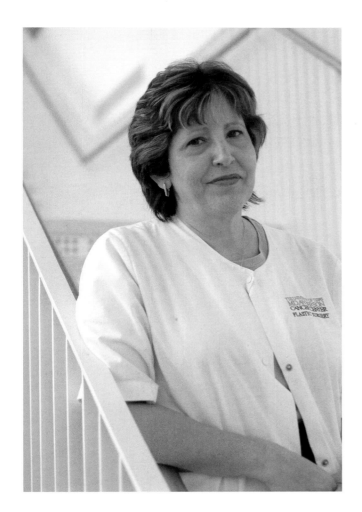

Callie Suniga, R.N.
Outpatient Clinical Nurse, Plastic Surgery Center
M. D. Anderson Cancer Center

When I came to M. D. Anderson to work as a nurse, I thought I was bringing with me my previous nursing experience to incorporate into the clinic. Little did I know that after working here for only nine months, I would be diagnosed with breast cancer.

My patients gave me support throughout my six months of chemotherapy and six weeks of radiation treatment. This experience definitely helped me to look at life and my patients differently. As a result, I can now add this to my personal experience and use it to support my patients who are just beginning their journey.

I work with two wonderful plastic surgeons here at M. D. Anderson, and, together as a team, we strive to create a positive experience for our patients. Breast reconstruction can be a lengthy process, but it is also a rewarding one both for the patient and the plastic surgery team.

HAIR & MAKEUP

We extend our deepest appreciation to professional make-up artist Athena Laster for donating her time, resources and artistic touch toward the making of this book.

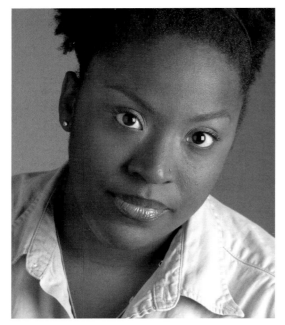

Athena Laster

Athena was born and raised in Houston, Texas. A graduate of Houston's Episcopal High School and HBCU, Hampton University, Athena displayed signs of promising artistic ability from an early age, choosing artists' canvases, oil paints and paintbrushes as her tools of trade. During her freshman year while preparing for the year-end ball, Athena discovered a new canvas . . . the face! It was then that she switched from oil paint to makeup and bought some softer brushes. Armed with Kevyn Aucoin's "Making Faces," Sam Fine's "Fine Beauty" and her new tools, Athena began to hone her skills in the art of makeup.

After graduating in 2000 with a Bachelor of Arts in Communications, she returned to Houston to work for MAC cosmetics. In this arena, surrounded by other gifted make-up artists, Athena was able to stretch her creative wings, working on every shape, shade and style of face. Athena credits her years with the company as a great learning experience. In 2003, she moved on to pursue her personal goal of being an independent professional makeup artist.

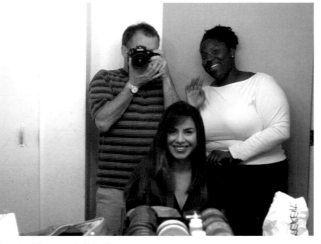

Jack, Athena & Martha

Athena and fellow makeup artist Teresa Chuck founded Divado! mobile makeup service. And, in 2004, she started "MAKEUP!!" a freelance service for commercial and editorial print, film and music videos. Her work can be seen in countless music videos and print publications, and this ferociously ambitious artist believes this is only the beginning. When asked what is next, Athena said, "I want to LIVE more, LEARN more and DO more!"

The future surely holds nothing but the best for this artist, who is always striving to better herself, her craft and her industry. Question: "Why ask a mortal? . . . When you can ask a GODDESS!" www.athenalaster.com

We also thank the following individuals for lending their talent and time to this project:

Tanisha "Tee" Burr, professional makeup artist & owner, www.makeupamore.com

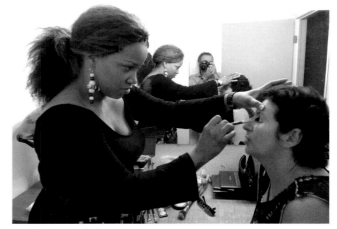

Tanisha & Emma

Shiwanna Archer, assistant volunteer coordinator
M. D. Anderson Beauty/Barber Shop Services

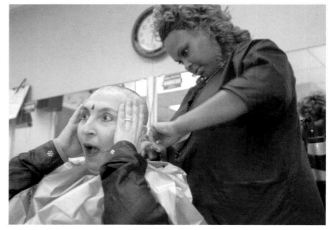

Shiwanna & Miss Josephine

DONORS

Rajani & Sophia Agnihotri	
April Ahern	In memory of Therese Roy
Jerry Alexander	In honor of Pam Alexander
Marquis & Rosemary (Oliva) Anderson	In memory of Maria T. Oliva & Dorothy I. Anderson
Emelia Appel	In honor of Natalie Faunda & Sophia Harasuk
Harvinder Arora	In honor of Josie Sethi
Bob Azimi	In honor of Josie Sethi
Mary W. Barrows	In memory of Thomas Chin
Anita & Dave Bille	In honor of Susie, Josie & Cathy & In memory of Grandma Bille
Molly Bobrow	In memory of Lori Mushovic-Halverson
	& Lori Summerford
Chad Borchgardt	In honor of Margaret Mallard
John & Kimberly Bowron	In memory of Ann Oppecard
Donna Brancifort	In honor of Josie Sethi
Ken & Patty Brown and Family	In memory of Josephine R. Robinson
Ruth & Al Buergermeister	In memory of John Buergermeister
Elizabeth M. Camp	In memory of Nita Beth Camp & Debbie Bohannon McKinney In honor of Lea Wade-Torres
Flo Carroll	In honor of Pink Ribbon Volunteers
Joe Caruso	In honor of Josie Sethi & Wayne Hardy In memory of Bob Reese
Dr. Saverio Caruso	In memory of Domenica Margaret Caruso

Kanwar & Kiki Chadha	
Dr. William B. Chan & Staff	In honor of Josie Sethi
Dennis Ming-Hong Chen Foundation	In honor of Josie Sethi
Don Clements	In memory of Shirley Richardson
Riddhi & Pankaj Desai	In honor of Josie Sethi & Jyoti Dalal
Shankar Deshmukh	In honor of Anita P. Deshmukh
Larry, Jim, Pamela & Maggan Dolan	In memory of Lyla Dolan
Cheryl & Pat Donlin	
Judy Epps	In honor of Beryl Bennett
Janet Ely	In memory of Ronda Goodier
Sudeshna (Sue) Fidora	In memory of Manoj Bhattacharya
Donna Fong	In memory of Cheryl Burguieres & Patricia Hanneman
Jo Frank	In honor of Sue McCallin
Jeannie Frazier	In honor of Josie Sethi In memory of Diane Schalles
Mimi & Jim Geihsler	In honor of Helen Geihsler & Debbie Rufo In memory of Debra Soduk, David C. Engle & cousin, Lina Gliozzi
Maike Miller George	In honor or Maike Miller George
Jackie Gilbreath	In memory of Billye Bell & Diane Duskin
Frank & Amy Gliozzi	In memory of Lina Gliozzi
Joseph Gliozzi	In memory of Michelina Gliozzi
Nancy Good	In memory of Barbara Newton Fanelli
Kurt & Nanette Goodenberger	In honor of Charolette Ciaraldi
Denise & Dana Goodman	

Gary & Laurene Grates and Family	In memory of Corinne Grates & Angela Giruzzi
JoAnne K. Gulliver	In memory of Gretchen Nakayama, Carolyn Beaman & Allison Grove
Lisa Hahn	In honor her mother, Ann Ditto & sister-in-law, Sally Ditto
Cindy & Henry Harrison	In honor of Judy Bloss
Denise Hazen	In honor of Betty Lou Sueman & Mary Bellos
Louis Helwig & Adam Helwig	In memory of Alicia Helwig
Rosemary Herron	In memory of Ronda Goodier
Randall & Anastasia Hobbet	In honor of Mary Hutchinson
Brenda K. Hoffman	In honor of stem cell research, Dr. Phil McCarthy & Dr. George Carrum
Brenda K. Hoffman	In honor of Toni Sinclair, angel to many
Brenda K. Hoffman & Toni Sinclair	In memory of Michelle Holmes, friend & oncology nurse
Jimmy Hoffman	In honor of Brenda K. Hoffman
Jeff James	In honor of Monique James
David E. Johnson	In memory of Mary E. Johnson
Vanessa & George Jurkovich	In honor of Lucille Farelli
Susanna Kane	In honor of Laura Mannetti
Mohan & Nishi Kashyap	In memory of Harish Chandra Kashyap & Sumitra Kashyap
Cecile & Ron Lavoie	In honor of Josie Sethi
Liz Lewis	
Sue Lewis	In memory of Marsha Ellen Hogg
Diane & James Littlefield	In memory of Erin Hennessey Hussey
"Glorious" Livengood	In memory of Mark Livengood

Lindsey & Beau Livengood	In memory of Mark R. Livengood
Ellen Lizotte	In memory of Esther Christine Ryan
Argelia V. Lopez	
Janet L. MacKenzie	In honor of Martha Remsen & Josie Sethi
Pat McWaters	In memory of Anna Beatrice Fisher (Mother)
Kelly Jo Myers-Madoian	In honor of all the Rosebuds members
Julia Maas	
Susan Medsger	In honor of Donna Parker
Alison Miller	In memory of Myrtle Miller
Sudhir & Chitra Minocha	
Joan & Steve Morgan	In honor of all cancer survivors
Josephine Sergio Muhlherr	In memory of Anthony & Joseph Sergio (brothers)
Mohan & Parvathy Nair	
John & Elizabeth Oliva Neidhart	In memory of Maria Oliva and Genevieve Neidhart
Martha Lucia Ocampo	In memory of Martha & Arturo Ocampo
Catherine Oliva	In memory of Caterina D'anna Napoli
Angelo & Frances Oliva	In memory of Giosofatto Vergara
Steven J. Palcko	In honor of Helen Patten Walsh
Claudette & Jack Peters	In honor of Josie Sethi
Patti & John Proach	In honor of Josie Sethi
Mary Raia	In honor of Josie Sethi In memory of Rosetta Navarro & Diane Waller
Pat & Ranjit Randhawa	In honor of Josie Sethi
Tony & Sally Romano	

Terri & Ed Roth	In memory of Cheryl Ebert
Catherine M. Sergio	In memory of Paul & Margaret Sergio
Robbie Clipper Sethi &	In honor of Josie Sethi
Davinder Sethi	In memory of Deborah Tall
Robert Lee Slaughter	In honor of Beverly Fuller Slaughter
Blane Smith	In honor of Kitty Smith
Emily Snyder	In memory of Charlene Brietzke
John & Cathy Soulliere	In honor of Yvette Soulliere & Peggy MacVarish
Jane & Bill Stangeland	
Marian Stanton	
Dr. & Mrs. Richard E. Stanton	
Rory Stanton	In honor of Nancy Maruyama
Mr. & Mrs. Thomas Steffan	
Jitty & Adip Thathy	In memory of Mr. Harcharan Singh Thathy (father) & Mrs. Rattan Kaur Thathy (mother)
Manmohini Thathy	In memory of Gurmukh Singh Sethi
Mariah & Cody Toscano	In memory of Frank Toscano
Rosie Toscano	In memory of Margaret Caruso
Kathy & John Unverzagt	
Dr. Sam T. Varghese & Staff	
Peter & Debra Violand	In honor of Ann Violand & Tommie Pippen
Janet Walsh	In memory of Maurice J. Walsh
Mark Welker	In memory of Mom, Wilma Welker In honor of Sis, Mitzi Seraphin
Marsha Yeager	In memory of Ronda Goodier

Richard A. Zansitis	In honor of Suzanne M. Mitchell
Maria Zappia	In honor of Josie Sethi
Stephanie Zerger	In honor of Merry Templeton, Eileen Chipperfield
	In memory of Alma Broussard & Effie Zerger

INDEX